Therapy Research
processes and practicalities

Jane Seale BSc, PhD
*Lecturer in Information and Therapy, University of Southampton,
Highfield, Southampton, UK*

Sue Barnard MSc, MCSP
*Lecturer in Physiotherapy, School of Occupational Therapy and Physiotherapy,
University of Southampton, Highfield, Southampton, UK*

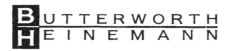

BUTTERWORTH HEINEMANN

OXFORD   BOSTON   JOHANNESBURG   MELBOURNE   NEW DELHI   SINGAPORE

Butterworth-Heinemann
Linacre House, Jordan Hill, Oxford OX2 8DP
225 Wildwood Avenue, Woburn, MA 01801-2041
A division of Reed Educational and Professional Publishing Ltd

A member of the Reed Elsevier plc group

First published 1998

British Library Cataloguing in Publication Data
Seale, Jane
    Therapy research: processes and practicalities
    1. Therapeutics – Research
    I. Title   II. Barnard, Sue
    615'.072

Library of Congress Cataloguing in Publication Data
Seale, Jane.
    Therapy research: processes and practicalities/Jane Seale, Sue
    Barnard.
    p.   cm.
    Includes bibliographical references and index.
    ISBN 0 7506 3435 9
    1. Physical therapy – Research – Methodology.   I. Barnard, Sue.
    II. Title.
    RM708.S43   98–27542
    615.8'2'072–dc21   CIP

ISBN 0 7506 3435 9

Typeset by AFS Image Setters Ltd, Glasgow
Printed and bound in Great Britain by Martins of Berwick on Tweed.

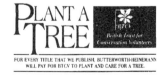

FOR EVERY TITLE THAT WE PUBLISH, BUTTERWORTH-HEINEMANN
WILL PAY FOR BTCV TO PLANT AND CARE FOR A TREE.

Contents

Preface

At the time of writing this book the authors have spent five years running the research methods course for undergraduate students at the Southampton School of Occupational Therapy and Physiotherapy. Therefore, this book has been written partly with students in mind. We hope that it provides them with a useful introduction to research. From an academic point of view we feel that students need to understand the process of research from initial idea to writing up. However, in talking about the process of research it is very easy to make things sound obvious and easy. They are not. Therefore from a practical point of view we wish to show students how research needs to be firmly bound in reality and the 'real world'. We also anticipate that this book will be useful for those qualified therapists who are embarking on their first 'research journey'.

This book incorporates a lot of examples, both real and hypothetical. The authors would like to make it clear that any names used in hypothetical examples are fictional and are not based on any real persons. Readers will also note that throughout the book the terms 'subject' and 'participant' are used interchangeably. On the whole, the term 'participant' is preferred as it indicates an equal relationship between the people providing and collecting the data. However, in some research designs and methodologies the term 'subject' is a more recognized or usual term.

Whilst we hope that this book will be useful to you, whether you are a student or a therapist, we do not expect it to be the only book or reference that you consult. There will never be a single book that will see you through all of your research experiences! That is why we have provided an extensive list of references and complementary reading for each chapter. This book will simply start you off on your journey and point you in the right direction.

Acknowledgements

We would like to thank the following people for inspiring and supporting us while writing this book: Fleur Kitsell and Rosemary Barnitt for allowing us time to write this book; Chris Davey, Judith Chapman and Rose Wiles for providing help with references and editing; Crissi Gallagher and Jani Grisbrooke for permission to use examples from their work; and finally, all the undergraduate students (past and present) at the Southampton School of Occupational Therapy and Physiotherapy.

1   What is research and why do therapists need to do it?

What is research?

If you were asked to define what research meant to you, then you may respond with phrases such as boring, exciting, rewarding, exhausting or frustrating. These phrases may reflect your personal response towards research. If you were asked to define what exactly research was, then your definition may have a different meaning to the definitions of other therapists.

THERAPY EXAMPLE

Cusick and Rotem (1994) conducted an exploratory study of how occupational therapy clinicians define research. They gave a questionnaire to 26 occupational therapy clinicians. The questionnaire presented four open-ended questions regarding research that were devised to elicit information about the respondents perceptions of the activities, behaviours and characteristics which constitute research. For example: 'A perplexed student asks you, "But what is research?" Write your answer here'. The responses were content analysed in order to develop categories of similar responses. Answers to the question 'But what is research?' revealed a variety of conceptual and operational definitions of research. Some focused on the outcome or product, e.g. 'finding a solution' or 'answering questions'. Others focused on research as a process, e.g. 'investigation'. Based on these responses, Cusick and Rotem constructed a composite definition of the term 'research': 'An orderly process of investigation, which produces new knowledge'.

EXERCISE

Ask your friends and colleagues to describe to you what research means to them. List all their responses. Can you identify responses that might fall into negative and positive categories? If you can, list all the positive responses in one column and all the negative responses in another column. If the responses do not appear to fall into negative and positive responses, are there other categories that you can identify which may help you to organize your data?

Most formal definitions of research centre on the notion that research is a method of science (Currier, 1990; Payton, 1988). Definitions tend to relate to the process of doing scientific research and use a language that we often associate with laboratories and experiments. Definitions include those of systematic, controlled, objective, empirical, replicable and reliable.

Generally the outcome of research is seen as the answering of questions and the provision of knowledge. It is argued by some that research also provides truth and the verification of beliefs. We will see later in the book how and why this argument may become a little complicated when we consider the possibility that there may be more than one truth or belief. In health care terms the outcomes of research are considered to be definition of best practice along with an improvement of patient care and service delivery (Bury, 1996).

Can therapists do research?

There are many common conceptions about research that can fuel an assumption that therapists cannot do research because it is too

Table 1.1   A comparison of the therapeutic and research process

Therapeutic process	Research process
Patient and referral agent present facts to the therapist in order to identify WHAT the problem is or might be.	Problem identification
Almost immediately the therapist begins to arrange these facts in his/her mind and construct explanations as to WHY the problem might exist.	Formulating hypotheses
The therapist tests these explanations by conducting initial assessments and formulating a treatment or intervention plan.	Hypotheses testing
When carrying out a treatment or intervention the therapist collects information as to the patient's progress and reactions.	Data collection
Information from treatments or intervention is then analysed in order to decide if the treatment was effective.	Data analysis
If the treatment was ineffective then the therapist will need to reformulate his/her ideas as to the cause of the problem or the best solution to the problem. If the treatment is effective there may still be a need to formulate an opinion as to what the next thing to do is. Furthermore, if the treatment is consistently effective the therapist may use it again as his/her first choice in the treatment of that condition.	Hypothesis reformulation
The therapist shares his/her results and clinical experiences with others.	Dissemination of information

difficult. Conceptions such as research produces extensive mathematical data or only a select few are in a position to understand the principles of research have been used to argue that therapists should not be expected to conduct research. To counter this argument, several people have argued that, by the very nature of their work, all therapists are researchers. Drummond (1996, p. xvi), for example, states that: 'The basic tools of the researchers are the basic tools of any therapist'. A comparison of the therapeutic process with the standard research process reveals many similar skills and tasks (see Table 1.1) Even if we manage to overcome one hurdle and persuade therapists that they have the skills to conduct research, the next hurdle is to persuade therapists that they might actively want to be involved in research.

Do therapists want to do research?

There has been a lot of evidence to suggest that therapists do not want to do research. Reasons for this are varied; Skelly (1996), for example, argues that physiotherapists are afraid of questioning common assumptions about their clinical practice. The most common reason for therapists not wanting to do research seems to be that they do not consider research to be a central part of their job remit. Research is for someone else to do and a 'real' therapist does not do research. These reasons (or excuses!) may reflect therapists' attitudes and opinions towards research.

THERAPY EXAMPLE

> Hicks *et al.* (1996) conducted an investigation of attitudes to research in primary health care teams. This study looked at four primary health care teams, each comprising a manager, a general practitioner, a practice nurse, a district nurse, a physiotherapist and a health visitor. The investigators found that when the team members were interviewed they tended to report positive attitudes about the role of research in their own health care practice. When the respondents were asked to complete a repertory grid designed to get at their deep-seated views the responses were contradictory. In particular, there was a prevalent view that research was a discrete activity that was not integral to each member's role.

Those therapists who have positive attitudes towards research and wish to be involved in the research process can often foresee benefits for themselves. These benefits might include gaining a feeling of accomplishment, receiving recognition from peers, having the ability to influence and spread ideas, and obtaining the opportunity to enhance career prospects and gain expertise in an area.

While there is a range of attitudes towards research, there is also a range of attitudes towards the role that therapists take in research. For example, Taylor and Mitchell (1990) described the role of consuming (implementing) research and collaborating in other people's research as a passive one. By creating a dichotomy of active and passive roles in research Taylor and Mitchell may be in danger of negatively portraying the roles of implementation and collaboration. There are some who see these roles as important and argue that not all of us need to do research ourselves provided we are willing to take on board the research of others. For example, Irene Illott in her 1997 Barbara Penn Memorial Lecture stated that: 'Research is done by some, facilitated by others and implemented by all'. An emerging opinion appears to be that therapists need to have research skills in order to do research of their own, to facilitate and collaborate with other people's research and to implement the findings of themselves and others. However, there is a growing acceptance that therapists do not necessarily have to be engaged in all aspects of the research process. Newham (1997, p. 6) argued that what is needed is 'an increased generalized research awareness in addition to a relatively small proportion of active researchers'.

Should therapists do research?

Argument and debate surrounding whether or not therapists should do research focuses on three main issues: raising our professional status, evidence-based practice and ownership of our knowledge base. We will consider each issue in turn.

Raising our professional status

There is a strong feeling that it is only through a continual examination of our knowledge bases that our professions can grow, develop, flourish and survive. Research offers therapists a real opportunity to determine the shape of their profession (Piper, 1990). The move to degree status, for example, with its emphasis on research dissertations, is argued to lend an academic and professional credibility to physiotherapy (Hicks, 1995; Newham, 1997). Research also provides a means by which other professions can learn from us and we can learn from them (Currier, 1990).

Evidence-based practice

For most of us, our treatments and interventions have often been based on intuition, familiarity, ritualistic behaviour, clinical judgement and historical precedent. There is often very little evidence to suggest that our practice actually works. There may also be evidence to suggest that our interventions are actually ineffective or dangerous (Hicks *et al.*, 1996).

There is a changing culture within health care delivery that places emphasis on the importance of accountability and effectiveness. One major consequence of this has been a move towards an evidence-based culture in which practice is justified on the basis of sound evidence. In a market economy such as that which exists within the British health system at the moment, services will not be purchased unless there is some evidence that the service is of good quality and has successful outcomes.

Evidence-based practice involves evaluating your own practice and utilizing the research findings of others. It is intended to provide a firm 'scientific basis' for improving services to patients. Delin (1994, p. 84) states:

'Nevertheless those who wish simply to practise their profession must have an understanding of the research process and the interpretation of research findings sufficient to enable them to keep abreast of current knowledge and to incorporate new and better procedures into their practice'.

The strong move towards evidence-based practice has signalled a move away from using therapies that have not been critiqued for scientific merit. Treatments are beginning to be defined as either standard or non-standard. For example, Harris (1996) identified five characteristics of non-standard therapies. One characteristic of non-standard therapies is that they fail to provide theoretical support based on current concepts and therefore lack scientific credibility. Another characteristic is the claim that they are effective for a broad range of diagnoses (a claim that should apparently provoke scepticism). However, the sands of evidence-based practice are still shifting and there is a current move back to the evidence base of clinical experience. Perhaps Sackett *et al.* (1996, p. 71) offer the best compromise:

'The practice of evidence-based medicine means integrating individual clinical expertise with the best available external clinical evidence from systematic research'.

Ownership of our knowledge base

A frequent reply to those of us who argue against research is 'if we don't do it, somebody else will do it for us'. For some this may not appear to be a problem. As long as it is not our personal responsibility to do the research, what does it matter? But, we would like to wager that those of us who visualize someone else doing the research, visualize a fellow therapist. If we all abdicate responsibility for research, then perhaps there won't be a therapist left to do the research!

In the current era of evidence-based practice it is unlikely that any health care system will allow a situation to occur where information is not collected in order to evaluate treatment and service provision. If therapists will not collect the data then other professions may be appointed to do so. Historically, it is not unusual for the therapeutic professions to rely on the research work of other disciplines such as medicine or psychology (Delin, 1994), so it may not seem inappropriate for these disciplines to provide us with the evidence for our current practice. There is a major risk, however, that the research questions posed by outside professionals will not have a specific relevance to our own models and practices. For example, in the field of evidence-based medicine, the only 'evidence' that has been considered acceptable is the evidence obtained from randomized controlled trials (see Chapter 3 for definition). It has been argued that for many areas of health care (including therapy) randomized controlled trials are unpractical or unethical. They also ignore or conceal important socio-political issues such as what the patient values. If we rely on researchers from other professions who see randomized controlled trial evidence as the only evidence worth having, then we run the risk of focusing our treatment solely on the disease or condition and not on the patient. This would appear to go against a lot of the values and principles of both occupational therapy and physiotherapy.

Changing expectations and practice

There are several suggestions for how we can change therapy expectations and practice to include more research activity. One argument is that we need to start from where we are and understand the current nature of therapy research in order to bring about a change in future research activity (Cusick, 1994). Another argument centres on changing our definitions of therapy practice to include research activity (Piper, 1991). Therapists are already beginning to identify gaps in research knowledge that need addressing through therapy research. For example, Tyrell and Burn (1996) identified that in the relatively new field of occupational therapy in primary care little research had been conducted into the health outcomes. In an attempt to identify health outcomes they conducted an evaluation of primary health care occupational therapy in a London health centre.

Whether we describe current practice, redefine old practice or identify information relevant to new practice, there is a changing expectation that therapists will engage in research in some way in order to provide the best therapy. As Newham (1997, p. 11) puts it:

'However, we must embrace the special features of physiotherapy in a positive manner and go forward with open minds to gain the knowledge necessary to know what constitutes best effect, for the sake of our patients, of ourselves and of our profession'.

Key points

1. Our personal definitions of research will vary. Formal definitions focus on the notion of research as a science.
2. The skills that therapists have place them in a good position to be a researcher.
3. Therapists have been reluctant to conduct research.
4. By getting involved in research therapists will raise their professional status, contribute to evidence-based practice and take ownership of their knowledge base.
5. There is a change in the expectations and practices of therapists regarding research.

References

Currier, D. (1990). *Elements of Research in Physical Therapy*. Williams and Wilkins.

Cusick, A. (1994). Collaborative research: rhetoric or reality? *Australian Occupational Therapy Journal*, **41**, 49–54.

Cusick, A. and Rotem, A. (1994). Definitions of research by occupational therapy clinicians: An exploratory study. *Australian Occupational Therapy Journal*, **41**, 99–114.

Delin, C.R. (1994). Research attitudes and involvement among medical students and students of allied health occupations. *Medical Teacher*, **16**, 83–96.

Drummond, A. (1996). *Research Methods for Therapists*. Chapman & Hall.

Harris, S.R. (1996). How should treatments be critiqued for scientific merit? *Physical Therapy*, **76**, 175–180.

Hicks, C., Hennessy, D., Cooper, J. and Barwell, F. (1996). Investigating attitudes to research in primary health care teams. *Journal of Advanced Nursing*, **24**, 1033–1041.

Illott, I. (1997). *Building bridges between research education and practice*. Barbara Penn Memorial Lecture, Southampton School of Occupational Therapy and Physiotherapy.

Newham, D. (1997). Physiotherapy for best effect. *Physiotherapy*, **83**, 5–11.

Piper, M.C. (1991). Physiotherapy and research: future visions. *Physiotherapy Canada*, **43**, 7–10.

Sackett, D.L., Rosenberg, W.M., Gray, J.A.M., Haynes, R.B. and Richardson, W.S. (1996). Evidence based medicine: what it is and what it isn't. *British Medical Journal*, **312**, 71–72.

Skelly, M. (1996). Research into reality. *Physiotherapy*, **82**, 428–431.

Taylor, E. and Mitchell, M. (1990). Research attitudes and activities of occupational therapy clinicians. *The American Journal of Occupational Therapy*, **44**, 350–355.

Tyrell, J. and Burn, A. (1996). Evaluating primary care occupational therapy: results from a London primary health-care centre. *British Journal of Therapy and Rehabilitation*, **3**, 380–385.

Complementary reading

Bury, T. (1996). *Introduction to Research*. Chartered Society of Physiotherapy. Chapter 2: Research: what is it and why?

Bury, T. and Mead, J. (1998). *Evidence Based Healthcare: A Practical Guide for Therapists*. Butterworth-Heinemann (in press).

French, S. (1993). *Practical Research: A Guide for Therapists*. Butterworth-Heinemann. Chapter 1: Introduction to research.

Hicks, C. (1995). *Research for Physiotherapists: Project Design and Analysis*. Churchill Livingstone. Chapter 1: Introduction.

Payton, O. (1988). *Research: The Validation of Clinical Practice*, 2nd Edn. F.A. Davis Company. Chapter 1: Basic concepts in research.

From research approaches to research questions

Characteristics and definitions of quantitative research approaches

In Chapter 1 we saw that definitions of research tend to equate research with a scientific method. The characteristics of a scientific method include those of objectivity, control and reliability. These characteristics tend to be associated with an approach to research called quantitative research. The characteristics of quantitative research are grounded in several assumptions:

1. Everything occurring in nature can be predicted according to reproducible laws.
2. Reality is tested by posing hypotheses that reflect anticipated answers to questions about cause and effect relationships.
3. The activity of investigating is perceived not to influence what the researcher is investigating.

These assumptions have led to research that tends to be conducted over relatively short periods of time in 'laboratory' situations where variables can be isolated. Such research may be considered to provide a singular, outsider's view of the context being studied. This approach to research has been used extensively in the natural sciences and has been used as the predominant paradigm in biomedical research.

THERAPY EXAMPLE

Drummond and Walker (1996) conducted a study that looked at the effectiveness of a leisure rehabilitation programme on functional performance and mood. The subjects were randomly allocated to one of three groups: a leisure rehabilitation group, a conventional occupational therapy group and a control group. Subjects in the leisure and conventional occupational therapy groups received individual treatment at home after being discharged from hospital. Assessments were carried out when the subjects were admitted to the study and three and six months after discharge from hospital. The assessor did not know which group the subject had been assigned to.

Possible reasons why quantitative research might be relevant to therapy stem from arguments about why therapists might need research skills. Such reasons include establishing legitimacy for many therapeutic procedures, demonstrating that specific procedures are valid when applied to individual clients in specific clinical environments and allowing measurements to be confidently quantified as opposed to guessed and approximated.

Characteristics and definitions of qualitative research approaches

For researchers interested in studying human behaviour, the use of research approaches guided and constrained by the laws of quantitative research causes considerable frustration. Out of this frustration has come an alternative approach to research called qualitative research. The assumptions of qualitative research include:

1. Individuals cannot be separated from the environment in which they function; the human experience needs to be studied as it occurs.
2. Reality is socially constructed by the individual, and thus multiple realities exist, not a finite number of objective truths.
3. An inductive process (discovery of general principles from particular facts or examples) generates a better understanding of unknown phenomena as opposed to deductive verification and testing of hypotheses.

These assumptions have lead to research that is conducted through an intense or prolonged contact with the field situation. Qualitative research can provide a holistic overview of the context under study in addition to offering an insider's view of the context or field. Such research also enables certain themes and expressions to be isolated. Miles and Huberman (1994, p. 1) offer a useful description of qualitative research:

> 'Qualitative data are sexy. They are a source of well-grounded, rich descriptions and explanations of processes in identifiable local contexts. With qualitative data one can preserve chronological flow, see precisely which events led to which consequences and derive fruitful explanations'.

Smith (1996) conducted a study looking at the working culture of physiotherapy assistants. This involved observing assistants over a period of a week for behaviours and interactions. Audio-taped semi-structured interviews were conducted in order to look at in depth feelings about working life and perceptions of qualified staff. The researcher also kept a reflexive diary throughout the study in which emergent ideas and feelings about the research were recorded.

THERAPY EXAMPLE

In considering the value of qualitative research in occupational therapy Robertson (1988) highlights two main difficulties with quantitative research. The first problem is that the objectives of a treatment programme are often difficult to express in observable terms, especially in rehabilitation programmes that are primarily concerned with the quality of life. The second problem is that quantitative research does not account for the unintended consequences that a hospital environment may impose. Robertson (1988, p. 345) argues:

> 'Considering that our field of expertise is to do with meaningful or purposeful activity in relation to the health of our patients or clients, it would seem that the qualitative approach should be an ideal one because phenomena such as meaning and purpose do not lend themselves readily to quantitative analysis'.

Physiotherapists argue that qualitative research is needed for a variety of reasons. Reasons such as the need to study the physiotherapist–patient interaction (Stone, 1991), the need to evaluate practice and thus help ensure high standards of care (Richardson, 1995) and the need to examine the multi-dimensional environment in which physiotherapists work and learn (Jensen, 1989).

We have identified and described two approaches to research and

Table 2.1   Differences between the quantitative and qualitative approaches to research

	Quantitative	Qualitative
Nature of reality	Reality is single and clearly defined.	Reality can be seen from a variety of perspectives and therefore a number of realities can exist.
Nature of the relationship between the researcher and the person or thing being researched	The researcher does not influence the subject: the two are independent of one another.	The researcher and the subject interact with and influence one another.
Influence of the context in which research takes place	Generalizations are made which are not specific to the context or time in which the research took place.	The researcher makes working hypotheses which are specific to the context and time in which the research is taking place.
Nature of the explanations as to why things happen	The cause of all effects can be identified and manipulated.	Things are caused by a number of factors all of which merge and interact with one another, therefore it is impossible to distinguish cause from effect.
Nature of the values attached to the research	Research is value-free because it is objective.	Research is value-bound and influenced by the values of the researcher.

called them qualitative and quantitative. There are other associated terms and descriptions of these two approaches. Terms and descriptions you may hear associated with quantitative research include positivism, natural science, objective, rationalistic, artificial and laboratory bound. Terms and descriptions that you may hear associated with qualitative research include phenomenology, social science, subjective, naturalistic, experiential and real world. These terms suggest that there is a strongly perceived difference between the two approaches. Guba and Lincoln (1982) define what they perceive to be the essential differences between the two approaches or paradigms. Their thoughts are summarized in Table 2.1.

These two different approaches to research are argued to influence the whole research process from purpose to data (Shepard *et al.*, 1993). For quantitative research the general purpose is to test, verify and explain. The purpose of qualitative research, however, is to describe and interpret phenomena. The research design of a quantitative study will be experimental to quasi-experimental as opposed to the non-experimental design of a qualitative study. The typical research methods of quantitative research include clinical trials and surveys. The typical research methods of qualitative research, however, include observation, interview and documentary analysis. The data that quantitative research generates tend to be numbers that can be subjected to statistical analysis. The data from qualitative research tend to be words or actions that are subjected to description, interpretation and comparison.

The need for both approaches in therapy research

Traditionally the two approaches to research have been presented as 'diametrically opposed'. Depending on your viewpoint, one research approach is superior to the other. This is a polarized argument that has stemmed from the beliefs and traditions that people bring to research. There is currently a growing acceptance that both research approaches have their place. Furthermore, both approaches can be seen to complement one another. This has led to calls to combine the two approaches where appropriate or to 'mix methods'.

Bryman (1992) offers a distinction of different ways and reasons why the two research approaches might be combined. These include the argument that the use of more than one research instrument to measure the main variables in a study offers validity to a project. Qualitative research can act as a precursor for the formulation of research questions and the development of measurement tools for use in quantitative research, while quantitative research can facilitate qualitative research by providing help in collecting qualitative data, for example by selecting cases for further study. Finally, qualitative and quantitative research can be combined in order to produce a general picture. Such a combination may allow a whole view of structure and processes and micro and macro levels, for example, combining observations and survey to provide a complete picture of a community.

Brannen (1992), however, warns against a naive integration of qualitative and quantitative approaches. She argues that if the purposes of the two approaches differ dramatically then the two data sets cannot be integrated to produce a single unitary picture.

THERAPY EXAMPLE

Demonstrating the need for a combined approach

Stewart (1996) reviewed the modalities that are used in the treatment of the hands of patients with rheumatoid arthritis: exercise, wax, and ultrasound. Stewart concluded that the results from the quantitative studies show marginal improvement with these modalities. Few researchers have addressed the individual and specific effects of the interventions and little is known about their long-term outcomes. The preventive strategies that could be employed in physiotherapy in the early and later stages of the disease remain unexplored. Stewart argues that qualitative research must be used to investigate such factors as compliance, interpersonal skills of the physiotherapist, patients' expectations and verbal encouragement. (See also Eklund, 1996.)

Going beyond current research approaches

Guba and Lincoln (1989) identified what they call three generations of evaluation: measurement, description and judgement. They call for a fourth generation of evaluation which they define as 'responsive constructivist evaluation'. Responsive in that the claims and concerns and issues of 'stakeholders' serve as the basis for determining what information is needed. Constructivist in that reality is constructed from a multitude of perspectives and sources. Stakeholders are people who are representative of the group being studied or potential users of the evaluation information. Stakeholders may belong to groups at risk or be open to exploitation and disempowerment.

The focus is moving away from the researcher deciding what and how to research, something that can happen in both qualitative and quantitative research. Instead, there is a move towards giving the participants and target populations more control over the whole research process.

Example of stakeholder involvement

Sample (1996) describes and evaluates a three-year research project that aimed to increase community participation by adults with developmental disabilities. She used a participatory action research method. This is a method whereby some of the people involved in the organization of the community under study participate actively with the researcher throughout the research process. For this study stakeholder involvement entailed assessment of need by everyone involved; developing potential solutions to problems; testing solutions to see if they are helpful; and accepting or rejecting the solutions. (See also Thomas and Parry, 1996 and March et al., 1997.)

Why do we need research questions?

Central to the idea of research is the notion that research attempts to answer questions. A research question influences the whole research process and provides a focus for the researcher. The nature of the research question will determine the purpose and approach of a research study. This in turn will influence the methods chosen to try and answer the research question. Once data has been collected, the researcher will attempt to determine whether his question has been answered and if not why not. Given the pervading influence of the research question, it is not surprising that most researchers agree that the most common reason for research failing is where there was not a proper question to start with.

Where do research questions come from?

In considering where research questions do not come from, Partridge and Barnitt (1986) argue that they seldom stem from 'intellectual exercises'. A research question needs more than creativity and inspiration to make it a good one. It is generally accepted that relevant research questions are derived from either clinical experience or the professional literature.

Clinical experience

Payton (1988) suggests that thoughtful reflection on your daily clinical experience may elicit doubts about the treatment procedures being used, or comments from patients or fellow workers may lead to a feeling of uncertainty and a desire to find out more. It is from this desire to find out more that research questions are born.

Research questions may come from a critical incident that happened in your practice or study that stimulates your thoughts and ideas. For example, imagine that you have observed one of your patients struggling to use the type of wheelchair they have been issued with. It is unwieldy and takes a lot of effort to move. Although the patient has tried to change their wheelchair they have been told that no alternative option exists. Your patient is disappointed and frustrated. As a therapist, the questions that may cross your mind might include: Does anyone have similar experiences? How satisfied are wheelchair users with their wheelchairs? How satisfied are wheelchair users with the wheelchair service? You could investigate these questions further in a number of ways. You could begin by looking at the literature in order to check whether your patient is alone in his/her problems. You may then try to get other people such as prospective funders and people in charge of the service interested in your idea. Finally, you may plan a study to look at users' and therapists' views regarding wheelchair assessment and provision in your region.

EXERCISE

Developing a research question from a critical incident
Part 1: Select an incident (it might be an event of a few minutes' duration or it might have taken 10 minutes or more) from your clinical experience which struck you as interesting or puzzling. Describe the incident briefly, but vividly, to a colleague or friend. With your colleague try to come to some explanation of the incident. Come to a view about your own position on the event and its significance. The following questions might help:
- What happened?
- What did it feel like?
- What made it happen?
- What did it mean?

- Why did it occur?
- What ought to happen now?

- What is it an example of?

Part 2: You have described your critical incident and attempted to explain it and apply meaning to it. Now, consider whether there are any questions that remain unanswered which you feel may be worthy of further investigation. List these questions and discuss with your colleagues.

The professional literature

Reading your professional literature may introduce you to conflicting theories and notions about the nature of health and how to treat it. This may stimulate research questions. You may doubt someone's findings and wish to explore their methodology further. You may disagree with the way someone has interpreted their results or the emphasis they have placed on certain findings. It may well be argued that our professional literature is not doing its job if it does not stimulate debate and questions!

Exploring the question

Having identified a possible research question, the next stage is to investigate the background of the question before you can move on to researching the answer with some confidence. You need to know whether someone else has had a go at answering your research question or whether someone has formulated your question in a better way. Your exploration will focus on both theoretical issues and methodological issues. The theoretical focus will look at what other people have thought concerning your question, while the methodological focus will look at what other people have done concerning your question.

This exploratory phase will be useful for the very final stages of the research process, writing up. A dissertation or article usually begins with some discussion of the background to the question, together with an overview of the existing literature (literature review). According to Bell (1987), the three main purposes of conducting a literature review are to examine how other authors have classified their findings, to examine how other authors have explored relationships and to examine how facts and relationships are explained. In conducting a literature review you need to firstly find the literature and secondly review what you have found.

Finding the literature

Muir (1993) gives a step-by-step guide to conducting a literature search. Firstly, you need to identify the scope of your topic by making sure you understand the objectives of the study and creating a list of key concepts and key words. Secondly, you need to define the parameters of your search. Parameters may include the date of publications you are going to search, the libraries you are going to use, the type of material (books, reports, web pages) you want and whether you will consider material written in a language other than English.

The third stage in finding literature is to choose your sources. You may wish to conduct a computer search using such computerized data bases as BIDS (Bath Indexing Data System) or Medline. Alternatively, you may prefer to conduct a manual search using subject catalogues, indexing and abstracting journals, current awareness services and citation indexes. Whichever source you use, you will need to keep a record of the information you have searched for and found. You may use an index card to record information about the books and articles you have found, such as author, title, place of publication and publisher. It may also be helpful to categorize the book or article you have found in some way. Categories may be things like qualitative to quantitative, positive or negative results or type of method used. You may also make a note of useful quotations.

The final stage of a literature search is to follow up any references that you cannot find by using interlibrary loan procedures and to make copies (remembering copyright laws) of any information that you need. The key to a successful literature search is finding relevant material quickly and avoiding getting bogged down (Bell, 1987).

EXERCISE

Finding the scope of the topic
Imagine you are on placement or at work; your supervisor tells you that in five days' time they wish to give a presentation on the following patients. You decide to go to the library to do some background reading. What key words are you going to use to focus your search?

Mrs Sarah Strong: Mrs Strong is 74 years old and lives at home alone. She was admitted to an acute hospital bed one week ago following a stroke. Her mood currently is one of depression as she feels she will no longer be able to enjoy her hobbies of gardening and painting when she gets back home.

Mrs Roberta Adams: Mrs Roberta Adams is 35 and has recently been diagnosed with rheumatoid arthritis. She lives with her husband and four children. She has been referred to physiotherapy for education and support regarding her arthritis.

David Downes: David Downes is a 12-month-old child who has been brought into the paediatric clinic by his mother because his development has been delayed. He is unable to sit independently, roll or crawl and his legs appear stiff. His mother is worried that David will never be normal.

Reviewing the literature

If we are to judge correctly what is and what is not appropriate to our own practice and research, we must be able to critically evaluate research reports (Parry, 1987). Parry (1987) and Drummond (1996) outline questions to consider when reviewing each section of a research article, from the abstract to the conclusion. Primarily their focus is on reviewing articles in order to decide whether they are good enough to publish or not. The purpose of reviewing articles here, however, is to decide whether your research question needs asking and, if so, how to answer it. Table 2.2 outlines how each section of a research report or article may help you to formulate a research question.

Table 2.2   Reviewing an article to formulate a research question

Section	Research review
Research question	How does this question compare with the question I want to ask? Same, different or related?
Introduction/ literature review	Did the authors conduct the study for the same reasons that I want to conduct my study? Do the authors refer to work that helps to place my research question in a theoretical and methodological context?
Method	Is this a method that I wish to use in my study? What are its good and bad points?
Results	Have the results answered my own research question? Do I need to bother conducting my own research?
Discussion	Do the researchers offer any discussion that may indicate whether or not my research question is worth investigating further?

Types of research question

Once you have conducted a literature review you may be ready to formulate a research question. As we have already indicated, the research question you set may give an enquiry a set purpose that will influence the specific design or plan of how the research will be conducted. Research questions can be exploratory, descriptive or explanatory. Exploratory questions seek new insights or look at phenomena or situations in a different way or with a different viewpoint. Descriptive questions attempt to portray an accurate profile of persons, events or situations. Explanatory questions seek to explain a situation usually in the form of causal relationships.

Examples of research questions:

Exploratory: Do occupational therapy students needs social skills training? Are there viable alternatives to ultrasound?

Descriptive: How do occupational therapy students react to three weeks' intensive social skills training? How do people with spinal cord injuries react to their rehabilitation regime?

Explanatory: Why is 1 minute of ultrasound more effective than 5 minutes? What causes people with spinal cord injuries to become depressed during a rehabilitation regime?

Refining the question

Whatever the nature of your research question it will need to be refined in order to ensure that it is well defined, important, relevant, measurable and ethical. Research questions can be rendered inappropriate for research because the answer is already known, the question is not of general interest or the question in unanswerable.

Refining your research question may help you to elicit a general aim for your research project from which specific objectives can arise. For example, if the aim of your study is to describe current paediatric occupational therapy services then you may have several objectives. Your objectives may include describing the patients being treated by occupational therapists and defining their conditions; describing the referral, review and discharge procedures of the service; examining the relationship that paediatric occupational therapists have with other health care staff; and describing the nature and range of treatments on offer.

From these aims and objectives, a research question or hypothesis may emerge. A hypothesis is a prediction about what will happen in a particular situation. It predicts the outcome of the study and is the only form of research question to which a statistical test can be applied.

Examples of hypotheses:
Children with cerebral palsy will be treated for longer periods by paediatric occupational therapists than children with Down's syndrome.
Fewer children from rural areas will be referred to the paediatric service than from urban areas.

Key points

1. Approaches to research may be quantitative or qualitative.
2. There is a need for both approaches in therapy research.
3. There may be occasions when it is appropriate to combine the two approaches.
4. Research questions emanate from clinical experience and the professional literature.
5. A literature review may help you to explore your research question.
6. Research questions can be exploratory, descriptive or explanatory.
7. Research questions often need to be refined in order to identify aims, objectives and hypotheses.

References

Bell, J. (1987). *Doing Your Research Project*. Open University Press.

Brannen, J. (1992). *Mixing Methods: Qualitative and Quantitative Research*. Avebury.

Bryman, A. (1992). *Quantity and Quality in Social Research*. Routledge.

Drummond, A. (1996). Reviewing a research article. *British Journal of Occupational Therapy*, **59**, 84–86.

Drummond, A. and Walker, M. (1996). Generalisation of the effects of leisure rehabilitation for stroke patients. *British Journal of Occupational Therapy*, **59**, 330–334.

Eklund, M. (1996). Patient experiences and outcome of treatment in psychiatric occupational therapy – three cases. *Occupational Therapy International*, **3**, 212–239.

Guba, E.G. and Lincoln, Y.S. (1982). Epistemological and methodological bases of naturalistic enquiry. *Educational Communication and Technology Journal*, **30**, 233–252.

Guba, E.G. and Lincoln, Y.S. (1989). *Fourth Generation Evaluation*. Sage Publications.

Jensen, G.M. (1989). Qualitative methods in physiotherapy research: a form of disciplined inquiry. *Physical Therapy*, **69**, 492–500.

March, J., Steingold, B., Justice, S. and Mitchell, P. (1997). Follow the yellow brick road! People with learning difficulties as co-researchers. *British Journal of Learning Disabilities*, **25**, 77–80.

Miles, M.B. and Huberman, A.M. (1994*). Qualitative Data Analysis: An Expanded Sourcebook*. Sage Publications.

Muir, M. (1993). How to plan and carry out a literature search. *Physiotherapy*, **79**, 781–782.

Parry, A. (1987). Guidelines to appraising research papers in journals. *Physiotherapy*, **73**, 375–378.

Partridge, C. and Barnitt, R. (1986*). Research Guidelines: A Handbook for Therapists*. Heinemann.

Payton, O. (1988). *Research: The Validation of Clinical Practice*, 2nd Edn. F.A. Davis Company.

Richardson, B. (1995). Qualitative approaches to evaluating quality of service. *Physiotherapy*, **81**, 541–545.

Robertson, L. (1988). Qualitative research methods in occupational therapy. *British Journal of Occupational Therapy*, **51**, 344–346.

Sample, P.L. (1996). Beginnings: participatory action research and adults with developmental disabilities. *Disability and Society*, **11**, 317–332.

Shepard, K.F., Jensen, G.M., Scmoll, B.J., Hack, L.M. and Gwyer, J. (1993). Alternative approaches to research in physical therapy: positivism and phenomenology. *Physical Therapy*, **73**, 88–101.

Smith, S. (1996). Ethnographic inquiry in physiotherapy research. 1. Illuminating the working culture of the physiotherapy assistant. *Physiotherapy*, **82**, 342–348.

Stewart, M. (1996). Research into the effectiveness of physiotherapy in rheumatoid arthritis of the hand. *Physiotherapy*, **82**, 666–671.

Stone, S. (1991). Qualitative research methods for physiotherapists. *Physiotherapy*, **77**, 449–452.

Thomas, C. and Parry, A. (1996). Research on users' views about stroke services: towards an empowerment paradigm or more of the same? *Physiotherapy*, **82**, 6–12.

Complementary reading

Bailey, D.M. (1991). *Research for the Health Professional*. F.A. Davis and Company. Chapter 2: Reviewing the literature.

French, S. (1993). *Practical Research: A Guide for Therapists*. Butterworth-Heinemann. Chapter 2: Developing research ideas.

Lincoln, Y.S. (1985). *Naturalistic Inquiry*. Sage Publications. Chapter 1: Postpositivism and the naturalistic paradigm.

Tesch, R. (1990). *Qualitative Research: Analysis Types and Software Tools*. Falmer. Chapter 3: History of qualitative research.

Williams, R.M., Baker, L.M. and Marshall, J.G. (1992). *Information Searching in Health Care*. Slack Incorporated. Chapter 2: The resources: putting them to work.

3 From research questions to research methodologies

Turning research questions into projects

Once you have decided on a research question, you need to identify the specific research methodology that will be appropriate for answering your question. If the research question is an expression of ideas and concepts, then the research methodology puts those ideas and concepts in an operational framework.

The selection of the research methodology follows naturally from the research approach. If you choose a qualitative approach then a certain set of methodologies are available to you; this set will be very different to the set available for a quantitative approach.

Qualitative research methodologies explored

Before providing an overview of qualitative methodologies it is necessary to issue you with some words of caution. In your reading around the topic of methodologies it is likely that you will become quite confused. For the qualitative approach problems with understanding and classifying the different methodologies stem from two main issues. The first issue is that terms which were once used broadly are now used to refer to a more specific methodology or purpose. For example, the term phenomenology was used in a broad sense as an alternative to or synonym for the term qualitative research (see Shepard *et al.*, 1993). The term is now used to refer to a more specific qualitative methodology.

The second issue is that people give different definitions and categorizations for the same research methodology. For example, in some texts people write about ethnography as if it were one singular methodology. Other writers will break ethnography down into different subcategories. These subcategories will be given different names and it can be difficult to equate the names that different people give to different categories.

Within qualitative research the source of information may be the spoken word, the written word or actions and behaviours. The source of information may influence the purpose of the methodology. Within qualitative research the purpose of the methodology chosen may be:

1. To identify characteristics.
2. To identify elements and explore their connections.
3. To determine patterns.

4. To ascertain meaning by identifying themes.
5. To ascertain meaning through interpretation.

Tesch (1990) makes the distinction between three different approaches in qualitative research. These distinctions illustrate how different purposes and sources will influence the methodologies. Tesch distinguishes between language-orientated, descriptive/interpretative and theory-building approaches. Language-oriented research approaches are interested in the usage of language and in the meaning of words. Descriptive/interpretative research approaches aim to gain insight into the human phenomenon or situation under study and to provide a systematic and illuminating way of describing the phenomenon. Theory-building research approaches try to do more than describe; they attempt to explain through the generation of theories.

We will now consider a range of qualitative methodologies, describe their characteristics, give examples where appropriate and outline advantages and disadvantages in their use.

Action research

Early examples of action research involved an external agent helping an organization to implement a change in response to an identified problem. The central notion was one of collaboration between the researcher and the participants. For example, Bond (1995) acted as an external change agent for an action research project in which a local authority wished to consider the needs of adults with serious physical disabilities who needed accommodation and full-time care.

Currently, action research has evolved into a methodology whereby an external agent or researcher is not always required. Practitioners are involved in the research processes that concern their own affairs. The notion of practitioner as researcher involves self-study and a desire to improve a situation. Action research is a very practical methodology with a strong problem-solving component. The practitioner identifies a problem during the course of his or her work and sees the merit in investigating it in order to improve practice. This approach is visualized to be ongoing or cyclical, with practitioners continually planning, acting and reviewing. Robson (1993) identifies the involvement of practitioners as a democratizing force as a principle characteristic of action research.

> Martlew (1996) describes an action research project in which a physiotherapist who worked at a Macmillan day hospice evaluated on-site physiotherapy. Patients' perceptions of the problems caused by their terminal illness, the relevance and benefit of physiotherapy and factors that contribute towards quality of life were investigated by the physiotherapist.

THERAPY EXAMPLE

According to French (1993) the value of action research is that it is a flexible and adaptable approach. A single practitioner or a group of practitioners can undertake it, the findings are implemented quickly, the research methods can be modified as research progresses and it may encourage more clinicians to take part in research.

Case study

If a researcher chooses to use a case study as a qualitative methodology, then they choose to concentrate on a single case. That single case may be a person, a community, a social group, an organization, an event or relationship. Sometimes a few individual cases are aggregated in one research report. A case study typically involves a detailed examination. Robson (1993) identifies that a case study can be exploratory or confirmatory. If a case study is exploratory it is trying to get some feeling as to what is going on in a novel situation, where there is little to guide what one should be looking for. If a case study is confirmatory it is based on previous work and is prestructured.

Allen and Skinner (1991) offer some characteristics of a case study. A case study places people's experiences in a specific social, economic and historical context. Its findings are not intended to be generalized to a wider population, but researchers may use selection criteria in deciding which case to study; it can be used to test theoretical propositions and it tends to use multiple methods such as documentary study, direct observation and/or interviewing.

THERAPY EXAMPLE

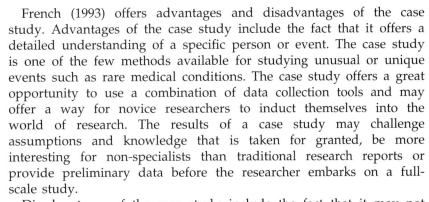

McKay and Ryan (1995) present a single case study of a second year occupational therapy student and an experienced supervisor. Both the student and the supervisor are asked to tell a story about one particular client they are working with. The stories were analysed in order to assess the benefits of narrative reasoning.

French (1993) offers advantages and disadvantages of the case study. Advantages of the case study include the fact that it offers a detailed understanding of a specific person or event. The case study is one of the few methods available for studying unusual or unique events such as rare medical conditions. The case study offers a great opportunity to use a combination of data collection tools and may offer a way for novice researchers to induct themselves into the world of research. The results of a case study may challenge assumptions and knowledge that is taken for granted, be more interesting for non-specialists than traditional research reports or provide preliminary data before the researcher embarks on a full-scale study.

Disadvantages of the case study include the fact that it may not offer an explanation for a certain situation, as it does not control for extraneous or confounding variables. On the other hand, others argue that case studies help us get at the casual links of real-life interventions. The data from a case study may not be generalizable to other cases as they are based on one person. Generalization becomes possible, however, if case studies are replicated.

Content analysis

Content analysis involves examining the content of communication and investigating what people communicate. A central idea in content analysis is that the words of the text are classified into a small number of content categories. The basic procedure is to design categories that are relevant to the research purpose and to sort all occurrences of relevant words or units into these categories. Content analysis can be quantitative or qualitative. An example of quantitative content analysis would be if the frequency of occurrences in each category were counted in order to draw conclusions.

For qualitative content analysis the usage of words is explored along with the range of meanings that a word can express in normal use. Target words are extracted with a specified amount of text before and after them. Then the researcher can group together words where the meaning is similar and establish how broadly or narrowly a certain term is construed. Word usage among groups of authors may be compared.

THERAPY EXAMPLE

> Reynolds (1996) analysed the essays of second year occupational therapy and physiotherapy students. The essays evaluated the impact of therapist communication skills on patient satisfaction, compliance and recovery. Analysis of essay content showed that students from both professions were generally aware of clients' cognitive needs and usually portrayed the therapist and patient as partners in effective treatment. There was a wide range of individual differences in the discussion relating to clients' emotional needs and the role of the therapists' listening and relationship skills in effective communication.

Discourse analysis

Discourse analysis or conversation analysis as it is sometimes called involves examining the process of communication and interaction, looking at how people communicate. Discourse analysis does not attend in any great detail to the context in which conversation is embedded. The analysis is done by breaking down the whole conversation into instances that can be compared with others in the same conversation. These instances are sorted in order to discover the structure of the language interaction in terms of regularities or to find linkages so that researcher can make 'assertions'.

Ethnography

Ethnography is a good example of how different people give different definitions and categorizations for the same research methodology. In some texts people will write about ethnography as if it was one singular methodology. Other writers will break ethnography down into different subcategories. These subcategories will be given different names and it can be difficult to equate the names that different people give to different categories. For example, Tesch (1990) makes a distinction between five main types of ethnography: structural ethnography, ethnoscience, ethnomethodology, ethnographic content analysis and classical ethnography. Muecke (1994), on the other hand, distinguishes between four categories of ethnography: classical ethnography, systematic ethnography, interpretative ethnography and critical ethnography. Most people when they are talking about ethnography are talking about conventional (classical or holistic) ethnography. However, it is important to explore the other subcategories in order to clarify our understanding.

Classical ethnography attempts to describe and analyse a culture by describing the beliefs and practices of the group and showing how various parts contribute to a unified, consistent culture. Classical ethnography has its roots in anthropology. Classical ethnography relies heavily on observation and, in some cases, complete or partial integration into the society being studied. This enables the researcher to share the same experiences as the subjects and therefore understand better why they acted in the way they did. The work in classical ethnography is generative; seeking to discover constructs and propositions. The analysis is conducted concurrently with data collection. The researcher reads the data in order to get a sense of the scope and topics, and then codes the data into categories that can be applied to segments of data. The appropriateness of the categories is checked and refined, and links between categories are sought.

Ethnographic content analysis is used to document and understand the communication of meaning as well as to verify theoretical relationships. It applies grounded theory to documents.

Ethnomethodology concentrates on how people make sense of 'indexical' expressions in communication. Indexical expressions are terms whose meaning is not universal but dependent on the context in which they are used. The ethnomethodologist is interested in aspects of daily life that are most taken for granted; in other words how people achieve implicit shared agreements with one another. Ethnomethodology looks at common sense everyday rules of social interaction. Trying to break what you think the rules are and observing people's reactions often does this. Ethnomethodology appears to be a very vague method with little written about it.

Sometimes called cognitive anthropology, ethnoscience involves developing models of the cognitive structure of a culture through an examination of its language. For ethnoscientists the end product is an expert system or data base to which anyone with an interest in the culture can refer. Material is elicited through a conversational interview. Most data come as responses to questions about 'naming units' (words and phrases) and the relationships between naming units. The first step might be to identify 'folk terms' and then to explore relationships between the folk terms and related terms. Relationships are depicted as diagrams and can be thought of as cognitive maps.

Structural or systematic ethnography uses classification of cultural terms and concepts in order to focus on interpersonal meaning. Structural ethnographers see their work culminating in the discovery of cultural themes within a culture. The end product is a verbal description of the cultural scenes covered. Material is usually obtained through the use of friendly conversation. The analytical procedures are quite similar to those of ethnoscience.

Schmoll (1987) considers how ethnography can be applied to physiotherapy. She argues that ethnography is well suited for studying physiotherapy in clinical settings because it can address systematically the types of therapeutic interventions we provide and how we interact with patients and others as we administer our treatments. Ethnography can help physiotherapists study interpersonal interactions, professional socialization, attitudes and values, patient compliance (concordance), teaching and learning, and the influence of environmental factors on the therapy process.

THERAPY EXAMPLE

Townsend (1996) collected data through observation, interview and documentary analysis over a six-month period. She used the data to describe the practice of occupational therapy in seven adult mental health day programmes and to answer the question: 'What are the possibilities and constraints for occupational therapists to enable the empowerment of adults who attend mental health day programmes?'. She used ethnography to show how the organizational context shapes occupational therapy practice.

The main advantage of ethnography is that it occurs in the natural setting. Baillie (1995) notes some difficulties in using ethnography. These include the fact that the researcher's presence as a participant observer may inevitably affect the social situation and disrupt natural behaviour. Writing while observing may be difficult and obtrusive, but if you write up afterwards you need to be quick or you forget! The observer may also experience role conflict, for example if they observe incorrect therapy practice or feel guilty for 'observing' rather than 'doing'. The ethnographer may feel too at ease and therefore too compliant or there may be a temptation to go native and abandon the research element in favour of the joys of participation. The result may be data that are limited or distorted.

Smith (1996) reflects on the impact that conducting an ethnographic study had on her and her research participants (physiotherapy assistants). Factors that she considered included the possibility that she had a biasing influence on the data collection and analysis, the need for the participants to trust her with the data, confidentiality problems with knowing some of the participants on a personal basis and problems with staying in researcher mode. There were also issues about controlling personal responses to situations. Smith concluded that through such methods as ethnography, physiotherapy could extend its body of knowledge and gain valuable insight into the beliefs and practices of the physiotherapy culture.

Focus groups

A focus group is a group interview that is focused on a particular topic and facilitated or co-ordinated by a moderator. This methodology is widely used in qualitative social science and market research and aims to capitalize on the interaction that occurs within the group. The focus group is useful for exploring poorly understood areas and attitudes and generating hypotheses.

Focus groups are often advocated in health care research in order to study consumer satisfaction and quality assurance. They may also be useful when studying health beliefs and attitudes. Sim and Snell (1996) identify four main applications of focus groups in physiotherapy:

1. Exploring patients' understanding, experience and attitudes towards health and health care – and inform health promotion services.
2. Evaluating health care through audit and consumer satisfaction.
3. Providing subjective data on the comparative impact of one treatment compared with another.
4. Studying practitioners' decision-making processes.

Focus groups are useful at any point in a research programme. Early on in the research process, focus groups can offer exploratory research where little is known about the phenomenon of interest. Other types of research that provide more quantifiable data may follow this. Later on in the research process, focus groups may be used after analysis of large-scale surveys in order to add depth to responses.

THERAPY EXAMPLE

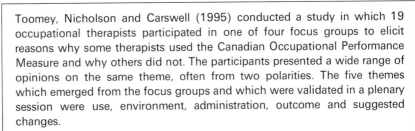

Toomey, Nicholson and Carswell (1995) conducted a study in which 19 occupational therapists participated in one of four focus groups to elicit reasons why some therapists used the Canadian Occupational Performance Measure and why others did not. The participants presented a wide range of opinions on the same theme, often from two polarities. The five themes which emerged from the focus groups and which were validated in a plenary session were use, environment, administration, outcome and suggested changes.

Stewart and Shamdasani (1990) consider the advantages and disadvantages of focus groups. Advantages of the focus group include the fact that large amounts of data can be obtained quickly at little cost. Using a focus group allows the researcher to interact with respondents to clarify responses, and follow up questions. Open responses also provide an opportunity for large amounts of rich data in order to get a deeper level of meaning. Focus groups allow respondents to react to and build on responses of other group members. The groups are flexible and can be used to examine a wide range of topics with a variety of individuals in a variety of settings. Focus groups are useful for collecting information from illiterate subjects and the results are often easy to understand.

Disadvantages of focus groups include the fact that the small nature of most groups limits generalization to a larger population. Generalizability is also limited by the potential bias that interaction between members brings. Problems may also occur if the researcher places more faith in the findings than is actually warranted. The open-ended nature of responses can also make interpretation difficult and risk researcher bias.

Grounded theory

Grounded theory is a methodology that allows theory to emerge from the data. Theories are derived from the fieldwork process, refined and tested during fieldwork and gradually elaborated into higher levels of abstraction towards the end of the data collection phase. Glaser and Strauss were the original proponents of grounded theory (1967) and distinguish between two procedures used in it: constant comparison and theoretical sampling. Constant comparison is a progressive clarification and definition of categories, while theoretical sampling involves deciding what data to collect and where to find it.

If a researcher chooses to use a grounded theory methodology, they choose to sort the incidents they find in their qualitative data into categories and then, through constantly comparing the content of them, to define the properties of the categories until they have taken on an abstract form. The result is a conceptual definition of the typical incident for a category. Conceptual categories are then related to each other. A grounded theorist is producing concepts that seem to fit the data.

Strauss and Corbin (1990) developed the coding process of grounded theory further. The grounded theorist may use open coding, where they look at the data line by line for empirical indicators that are actions and events. They ask themselves 'what category does this incident indicate?' and provide a code name for the category. The grounded theorist needs to continually verify that each code really does fit the data.

Once the researcher has become sure of a category they may engage in axial coding, which is intense analysis done around one category at a time. This results in cumulative knowledge about relationships between that category and other categories, along with knowledge about subcategories. At this point selective coding begins, whereby the researcher limits coding to those codes which significantly relate to the core codes in order to obtain a complete theory.

Bryman and Burgess (1994) argue that the influence of grounded theory has been two-fold. It has alerted researchers to the desirability of extracting concepts and theory out of data and has informed researchers of the use of different types of codes and their role in concept creation. Stern (1994) argues that grounded theory as a method is being eroded. She gives two reasons for this: arguments surrounding a perceived difference between Glaserian and Straussian methods of grounded theory (see Table 3.1) and investigators manipulating data in a haphazard way under the guise of grounded theory due to a lack of guidance or original reference material ('minus mentoring'). According to Stern, this has led to a muddling of methods, whereby researchers are mistaking grounded theory for other methods such as content analysis or phenomenology.

Because grounded theory can be seen as half art, half science a description of how to do it has become quite elusive. In some sense it is probably not possible to learn grounded theory from a book; you probably need to watch and learn from a grounded theorist in action. Strauss and Corbin (1990) have attempted to counteract arguments that grounded theory is too loose and have perhaps focused more on the science of interpretation, whereas Glaser focused on the art of interpretation.

Table 3.1 Differences between Glaserian and Straussian grounded theory

Glaser	Strauss
Glaserian grounded theory would be expected to be immediately applicable to those who shared the problem under study.	Straussian grounded theory does not emphasize applicability.
Glaser argues for allowing the theory to emerge.	Strauss has become quite prescriptive with his codified operation.
Has a focus on 'What do we have here?'.	Focuses on the 'What if?' question.
Allows the data to tell their own story.	Looks at every possible contingency whether it appears in the data or not.

Hermeneutics

Hermeneutics is similar to phenomenology but used on written texts. A singular event is understood by reference to whatever it is a part of. The analyst moves back and forth between individual elements of the text and the whole text in many cycles. The historical context in which the experience takes place is also considered.

Life history studies

Life history studies follow the development of events and experiences over time. Documents can be used in order to allow the researcher to travel further back when trying to gain insight into how our current reality has been negotiated and constructed over time. Alternatively, or in addition, an oral history can be taken. Using oral histories is the practice of eliciting memories from people in order to capture a past era or reality. In their true sense life histories start at a current time and look backwards. Life histories are used prospectively where a researcher starts at a current time and documents everything that happens from that point forward until a dedicated cut-off time.

Larson and Fanchiang (1996) argue that life history studies can provide occupational therapists with a better understanding of the complexities and contexts of clients and their experiences of the therapeutic process. They can provide the therapist with a view of the clients' daily occupations, routines, family relationships and socio-cultural influences. This method would seem to reflect nicely the humanistic roots of occupational therapy.

THERAPY EXAMPLE

Blanche (1996) used a life history study to examine the story of a mother who has a daughter with disabilities. The data were collected over an 18-month period from interviews, participant observation and review of records. Analysis focused on the coping strategies of the mother and the health care providers.

Phenomenology

Phenomenology derives from the Greek word phenomenon which means 'to show itself', to put into light, to make something visible. Phenomenology attempts to discover the essential meaning of human endeavours, to get at the meaning of an experience. Phenomenology is the study of the ordinary world and how people experience their world. In order to gain access to the experience of others, phenomenologists collect intensive and exhaustive descriptions from their respondents. These descriptions are submitted to a questioning process in which the researcher is open to themes that emerge. A theme is a topic, statement or fact. Finding commonalities and uniqueness in these individual themes allows the researcher to crystallize the constituents of the phenomenon. The result is a description of the general structure of the phenomenon studied.

The phenomenological researcher emerges themselves in the data, reading and rereading them. They look for meaning units or material

Table 3.2 Distinguishing between phenomenology and grounded theory

Phenomenology	Grounded theory
Derived from a philosophical tradition.	Derived from a sociological perspective.
Describes psychological realities by uncovering the meaning of lived experience.	Explains social or social psychological realities by identifying processes at work in the situation being studied.
The researcher does not use previous experience or knowledge.	The researcher uses previous experience and knowledge to influence his/her ideas and assumptions about the situation being studied.
The data come directly from informants who have lived the reality under investigation; the process 'borrows other people's experiences'.	Information about social processes is inferred from observations and interviews.
Sampling is purposive; informants are chosen because they have lived the experience being investigated.	Sampling is selective, selecting different data sources in order to discover variations in a situation.
Data analysis occurs after data collection.	Data collection and analysis occur concurrently and are based on a constant comparative method.
Validity depends on the extent to which the study truly reflects the essence of a phenomenon as experienced by the informant.	Validity depends of the usefulness of the theory that has been generated.

that relate to the phenomenon under observation, they restate the content or theme by summarizing or transforming, and then cluster similar meaning units together or give a descriptive statement of the themes.

THERAPY EXAMPLE

> Hasselkus and Dickie (1994) sought to understand the nature of the experience of doing occupational therapy. In order to do that they asked occupational therapists to think back over their practice and describe a very satisfying experience and a very dissatisfying experience. The task was to keep the therapists in the experience and not distanced by giving thought about the experience. From those experiential narratives Hasselkus and Dickie derived dimensions of the lived experience of doing occupational therapy.

Baker, Wuest and Stern (1992) argue that phenomenology and grounded theory are two methods that are often confused and that the differences between them can be blurred (see Table 3.2).

Overview of qualitative methodologies

Whatever qualitative methodology you choose as a researcher, there will be some common elements that influence what you do. Tesch (1990) offers a summary of qualitative methodologies. While the analysis process is systematic and comprehensive it is not rigid. There is no one right way to manipulate qualitative data and the procedures are not mechanistic. In addition to categorizing and sorting, attending to data includes a reflective activity that can guide the process. The result of using a qualitative methodology is argued to be a kind of 'higher level of synthesis'.

Quantitative research methodologies explored

In order to distinguish between different quantitative research methodologies a distinction is often made between experimental and quasi-experimental research methodologies. In experimental methodologies causal relationships are explored and predictions tested by manipulating one variable (independent variable) and observing changes in another variable (dependent variable). In addition to manipulating the independent variable, the researcher attempts to keep all factors that might confound or influence the results constant. In quasi-experimental methodologies researchers still attempt to manipulate independent variables but have less or no control over confounding variables and are unable to assign subjects to groups. Examples of experimental methodologies include the randomized controlled trial, and cross-sectional and longitudinal studies. Examples of quasi-experimental methodologies include the single subject design, clinical trials, time series design and correlational studies.

Randomized controlled trial

The randomized controlled trial (RCT) is often called the 'true experiment' or independent subject design. This methodology involves the random assignment of subjects to groups or conditions. Random assignment significantly reduces the likelihood that any extraneous difference between the subjects can account for differential performance on the dependent measure. The conditions for a randomized controlled trial are that the treatment group(s) experiences the independent variable (intervention or treatment) while the control group does not experience the intervention or treatment. Typically researchers may employ a pretest post-design, whereby measurements are taken on the dependent variable before and after intervention.

THERAPY EXAMPLE

> Burridge *et al.* (1997) describe a randomized controlled trial of the Odstock Dropped Foot Simulator (ODFS), a peroneal stimulator used to correct dropped foot during walking. A sample of 32 chronic hemiplegic subjects were randomly assigned to a treatment and control group. Both treatment and control group received a course of 10 physiotherapy sessions during the first four weeks of the trial period. The treatment group used the stimulator as part of the physiotherapy sessions and independently each day, as they found useful. Both groups received the same amount of therapy contact time. The treatment group continued to use the stimulator for the 12-week period.

Advantages of randomized controlled trials include the fact that they control for all confounding variables and allow for rigorous statistical testing. Disadvantages centre on the fact that it is a difficult method to execute in the real world of health care. For example, it may not be practically possible to randomize subjects into treatment and control groups. In addition, it may not be ethically acceptable to deny a subject the treatment by placing them in the control group.

Cross-sectional studies

Cross-sectional studies produce a snapshot of a population at a particular point in time. They investigate different groups of individuals at one particular point in time. Through sampling techniques it is possible to get a group of subjects (made up of different individuals) who are a representative cross-section of a population. Cross-sectional designs enable the researcher to gather information from a manageable number of subjects and to draw inferences about the population from which the sample was drawn.

The advantages of cross-sectional designs are often considered by comparing cross-sectional with longitudinal studies. For example, in cross-sectional designs the data are collected only once and therefore there is less risk of participants dropping out. It is also considered easier to find volunteers for a cross-sectional study than a longitudinal one as it takes up less time. Disadvantages of the cross-sectional study centre around the fact that it is difficult to make causal inferences because the same people are not followed through and the study takes place at one point in time.

Longitudinal studies

Longitudinal designs attempt to examine events or traits of a variable over a prolonged period of time. Measurements are taken from subjects at intervals over a set period. The information is of great value when interest is centred on changes that occur over time.

THERAPY EXAMPLE

> Westbrook and McIlwain (1996) conducted a five-year follow-up study of 176 people with post-polio syndrome. They compared experiences of anxiety, uncertainty, depression, helplessness and anger over time and found that feelings of anger had persisted over the five years, while feelings of anxiety, uncertainty, depression and helplessness had decreased. (See also Atkinson *et al.*, 1995.)

Two main disadvantages of longitudinal studies are that they tend to suffer from a loss of research participants as time goes by and they also tend to use relatively small subject numbers which may influence the researcher's ability to generalize the findings to a wider population. The major advantage, however, is the ability to map changes across time.

Single subject design

In this approach only one subject is studied as opposed to groups of subjects. Single subject designs are used to explore the effects of the independent variable on the behaviour of a single subject. Currier (1990) identifies three characteristics of single subject designs: the dependent variable (subject's performance) is repeatedly measured across time; the subject (participant) serves as his or her own control when comparing performances before and after treatment; and the multiple measurements provide some evidence of treatment effectiveness.

Single subject designs enable the observer to examine changes in subject performance as they occur, and with several data points the observer can predict future performances. Single subject designs are also called interrupted time series designs because measurements are repeated at specific time intervals. There are several single subject designs that can be executed. Each design offers a different combination of treatment (B, C) and baseline (A). A baseline gives a measurement with which later performance can be compared in order to assess progress (between five and 20 measurements are needed to give a clear picture of a subject's level of functioning).

In an ABA design, the subject's performance is measured on a baseline and then a treatment session is introduced in order to test whether performance changes. A second baseline is used to test whether performance returns to its pretreatment level. In an ABAB design, after an initial baseline, an appropriate treatment can be introduced, during which measurements of performance can be taken over a number of treatment sessions. The treatment will then be discontinued. Performance is measured on a second baseline in order to make comparisons with performance during treatment. The treatment is then repeated. An ABCB design can be used to counteract the placebo effect when the treatment phase is withdrawn.

The key to successful single subject designs is presenting the interventions in an unbiased manner and assessing outcome using a valid unbiased procedure.

Data from single subject designs are usually plotted on a graph and underlying trends demonstrated by curve-fitting techniques such as the split middle method. With this method the line of best fit is plotted for the baseline data and extended into the intervention phase, suggesting a predicted linear trend in each phase. This method lacks precision when the number of data points is small and may over-accentuate improvements in conditions which have a tendency to remit. Statistical tests such as *t*-tests and analysis of variance can be used but these were developed for use with group studies and are based on assumptions about the data which may not apply to a single case.

The advantages of the single subject design are often considered by comparing it with the case study method. For example, Cole (1991) argues that single subject research designs should be used in preference to case study methods, which he argues are essentially impressionistic and limited in terms of empirical validity. Gill, Stratford and Sandford (1992) suggest that single subject designs will help to close the gap between clinical research and clinical practice. This is because they can provide a more realistic representation of patient–therapy effects (measurement outcomes can be customized to each patient), and they can be used as a therapeutic effectiveness decision-making aid and to determine the cause of an adverse reaction.

Problems with the single subject design centre on the argument that the ABAB design and its variations may not always be appropriate in therapy research. Bithell (1994) outlines three major problems with using baselines. Firstly, it may take a long time to establish a baseline since data should be collected until consistency is achieved. Therapists may not have enough time to establish a baseline before they have to give treatment. Secondly, there may be problems with rising baselines in those conditions that have a natural tendency to improve (performance in baselines is expected to be worse than in treatment phases). Thirdly, the frequent testing and measurement required by this design might alter behaviour and increase the effects of error. In addition, once treatment has begun it may not be possible to revert to the baseline again (due to ethical reasons or because once an ability has been acquired or progress has been made it may not be possible to undo the progress or unlearn the ability).

Another frequent argument made against the single subject design is that it is difficult to generalize the results from one individual to others who may differ in a number of ways. While this may be true, it is also true of group comparison studies. Given the heterogeneity of patient groups it may be difficult to determine which characteristics of an individual patient meant that improvement could be made with the treatment.

| Group 1 | Test | Treatment | Test | No treatment | Test |
| Group 2 | Test | No treatment | Test | Treatment | Test |

Figure 3.1 Cross-over design.

THERAPY EXAMPLE

Hartveld and Hegarty (1996) tested the hypothesis that frequent weight-shift practice with feedback from a computer improves standing balance in children with cerebral palsy by using a replicated AB design with four children. Standing balance was tested twice weekly throughout the baseline and the treatment period (computerized feedback).

Clinical trials

Clinical trials can be seen as an attempt to use experiments in the real world of the health care setting. Clinical trials may be used where it is deemed impossible to randomly allocate subjects into experimental and control groups. They may also be employed where it is considered unethical to withhold a treatment from a control group. For example, in a cross-over design all groups of subjects have an opportunity to receive treatment at some time but not necessarily in the same order (see Figure 3.1).

THERAPY EXAMPLE

Protas *et al.* (1996) report a study which compared the aerobic capacity of individuals with Parkinson's disease (treatment) with that of individuals without Parkinson's disease (control group). Randomization could not be employed here because the researchers needed to force one group to have a certain characteristic, i.e. all had Parkinson's disease.

Time series design (cohort design)

With a time series or cohort design one group of subjects (cohort) is investigated at one point in time and another group of participants at another point in time (see Figure 3.2).

Time 1 (1997)	Time 2 (1998)
Group 1	Group 2
Treatment 1	Treatment 2

Figure 3.2 Time series design.

Table 3.3 Hypothetical scores on the Bartel and AMPS assessments

Participant	Score on Bartel Index	Score on AMPS
1	34	23
2	22	11
3	56	64
4	47	36
5	69	75

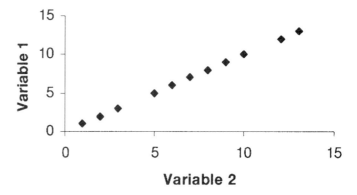

Figure 3.3   Positive correlation.

Correlational studies

Correlational studies do not attempt to manipulate independent variables or look at cause and effect relationships. Instead they attempt to investigate relationships or associations between dependent variables. The purpose of a correlational study is to estimate the extent to which variables co-vary or relate to each other. For example, we may take a group of five participants and for each participant measure their Bartel Index and AMPS score (see Table 3.3). Scores can be taken from the same individual as in the example or they can be logically paired, e.g. mother–daughter. The data may involve two scores on the same test or scores on two different tests. Correlations can be positive or negative (see Figures 3.3 and 3.4). A positive correlation can be obtained in two scenarios. The first scenario is where participants score high on one measure and score high on another separate measure. The second scenario is where participants score low on one measure and low on another measure. A negative correlation will be obtained when participants score high on one measure but low on another.

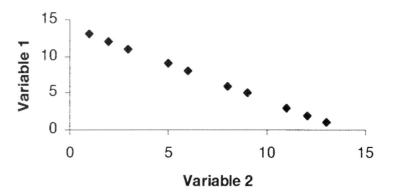

Figure 3.4   Negative correlation.

Correlational studies can be used as a rather broad search for principles upon which more specific experimental research can be built. Or they can be used with a very specific question or prediction in mind. Correlational studies are used to validate measurement tools and to investigate test–retest reliability.

Overview of quantitative methodologies

Therapists have been attempting to use quantitative methodologies for some considerable time. The success of their attempts, however, seems to be limited. For example, Pollock *et al.* (1993) conducted a review of the rehabilitation literature and concluded that there were very few well-designed and reliable studies in this area. Common weaknesses included lack of comparable controls, lack of adequate numbers, lack of appropriate outcome measures, lack of definitions of rehabilitation, failure to control for placebo effects and a lack of generalizability. The solution that Pollock and colleagues suggest is for more multi-centre clinical trials.

The dilemma for therapists attempting to conduct quantitative research is that of achieving a 'controlled approach' in the real world of health care. Grieve (1993) argues that some research trials in physiotherapy have not been 'fair' due to a lack of experimental control. She argues that such deficiencies may lead to professional practices being unjustifiably condemned.

EXERCISE

Take one of the two questions below and decide how you as a researcher would try and answer that question.

1. How effective are community mental health services for people with schizophrenia who have been discharged from hospital for over a year?
2. How effective is computer-supported education in reducing hospital admissions for asthmatic patients?

Mixing methodologies

There are two factors that influence our choice of methodologies. The first factor is our philosophical beliefs about the appropriate foundations for the study of society. The second is our technical beliefs about the appropriate methods for the study of society. The application of these two factors can lead to a conflict between qualitative and quantitative methodologies. Corner (1991) considers the conflict between qualitative and quantitative methodologies in nursing research and offers some advice that can apply to therapy research. She notes that a bipolar view of nursing research has arisen out of a desire to be accepted by more 'established' scientists. Corner (1991, p. 720) argues that 'new' disciplines such as nursing cannot afford to divide on the grounds of philosophical approaches to research.

'They need to develop new confidence, free from the constraints of sitting on one side of the fence or another, in order to explore the unique area of health care encompassed by nursing, in all its complexity'.

Research studies are not always purist in their application of different research philosophies. For example, many qualitative studies imply some form of measurement in their use of terms such as frequency, proportion, smaller and larger, while quantitative studies often incorporate participants' impressions and opinions verbatim. In reality, few studies are strictly quantitative or qualitative.

Brewer and Hunter (1989) outline a multi-method approach to research and argue that its fundamental strategy is to tackle a research problem with a range of methods that have non-overlapping weaknesses in addition to their complementary strengths. In considering the conflict between qualitative and quantitative methodologies, Parry (1991) argues that physiotherapists need to make more appropriate use of the whole range of methods available to them in order to evaluate clinical change, outcome from treatment and cost-effectiveness. Triangulation and the Delphi technique offer us a way of mixing methodologies.

Triangulation

The term triangulation is used to refer to combining different methods and techniques in various ways to study the same phenomenon. There are several different forms of triangulation. Data triangulation involves gathering different data about the same phenomenon. Theoretical triangulation involves using different perspectives to analyse the same set of data. Methodological triangulation involves using two or more methods of data collection in a single study, while investigator triangulation involves using different researchers to collect data at different stages in the research.

Methodological triangulation rests on the assumption that all methods have strengths and weaknesses, and the weakness of one method can be counterbalanced by the strength of another. Factors to take into consideration when thinking about using methodological triangulation include making sure the research question is clearly focused, and that the methods chosen are complementary and appropriate for the nature of the phenomenon being studied. It is recommended that continual evaluation of a triangulation approach should be undertaken during the study.

Corner (1991) and French (1993) offer advantages and disadvantages of triangulation. Advantages include the fact that it offers a flexible and in-depth approach. Triangulation may be useful when researching complex issues and can help to break down divisions between research perspectives. Disadvantages of triangulation include the considerable time and money required when combining different approaches. In addition, the investigator needs a broad knowledge-base and an ability to cope with a complicated design and there are few guidelines on how to combine numerical and textural data.

The Delphi technique

The Delphi technique takes its name from the Greek god Apollo Pythias. As master of Delphi, Apollo Pythias was known for his ability to predict the future. The Delphi technique can be utilized to collate and analyse the opinions of experts in a specialized field. This is usually achieved by sending sequential questionnaires to a selected group of people. The first questionnaire sets out to gain a response to a broad subject and the subsequent questionnaires are built upon the responses of the preceding questionnaire. It may take three to five rounds of questionnaires before consensus is reached.

Key characteristics of the Delphi technique are:

1. A panel of experts is used as the source of the respondents.
2. The exercise is usually a written one using sequential question-naires.
3. The aim is to produce a consensus of opinion.
4. The members of the panel and the origin of statements are not identified.
5. The statements from previous questionnaires are fed back to respondents.
6. The panel members will be given a summary (usually statistical in nature) of the results from previous rounds.

The success of the Delphi technique depends on allowing sufficient time for the questionnaires to be posted, returned and analysed, on members of the panel having good written communication skills and on panel members being motivated to take part.

The Delphi technique is not restricted to questionnaires and can therefore facilitate a mixed methodology approach. Studies have been reported that use interviews for the first round and follow up with questionnaires. Computer technology such as the Internet can also be used to enable a more instant sharing of information and immediate voting to take place (Beretta, 1996).

The Delphi technique may employ quantitative or qualitative methodologies. The qualitative approach of a Delphi study will concentrate on exploration while the quantitative approach relies typically on summarizing ranking statements in order of preference or priority. In addition to forming studies in their own right, this technique can also be used as a component part of a wider project.

THERAPY EXAMPLE

Barnard (1992) reports a Delphi study that she conducted for Wessex Regional Health Authority in order to identify health care needs of people with disabilities. In Round One, Questionnaire A was sent to disabled people, carers and representatives of voluntary bodies, charities and self-help groups. Questionnaire B was sent to clinicians, managers and medical specialists. Results from Round One were analysed to produce a list of identified problems. These problems were put in a second questionnaire and sent to all the original participants, who were asked to prioritize the categories of problems in order to importance and perception of need. (See also Dawson and Barker, 1995 and Miles-Tapping et al., 1990.)

Advantages of the Delphi technique include:

1. It utilizes a large number of opinions.
2. It avoids domination of the 'committee process' by one person; each participant has an equal voice.
3. People do not have to take public stances which they may find difficult to abandon later, and it avoids problems of conformity and risky shifts.
4. It reduces interviewer/observer bias.
5. It is relatively cheap.
6. It is likely that the information gained will be valid in that it will be relevant to the research question.

Despite these many advantages the Delphi technique has been criticized for its lack of 'methodological rigour'. For example, individuals may be influenced to conform because consensus views are fed back to each member. The study may also fail to get a representative sample of experts. Different panels with similar expertise may produce different results (lack of reliability) and the validity of the results may be influenced by the response rates. In addition there is little agreement on the optimum size of panels or on what constitutes 'consensus'. Jones and Hunter (1995) argue that the existence of a consensus does not mean that the 'correct' answer has been found. The Delphi technique has an equal chance of producing collective ignorance as well as collective wisdom.

From methodologies to methods

This chapter has sought to distinguish between the different methodologies that can be employed depending on whether you are adopting a qualitative or quantitative approach to research. For each methodology there are certain data collection techniques or methods that may be appropriate. These include the use of standardized assessment tools, observation, interviews and questionnaires. These methods will be explored in more detail in following chapters.

Key points

1. The selection of a research methodology will be influenced by the chosen research approach.
2. There is a range of qualitative research methodologies.
3. There is a range of quantitative research methodologies that may be experimental or quasi-experimental in nature.
4. There may be occasions where mixing methodologies is appropriate.
5. Triangulation and the Delphi technique allow you to mix methodologies.

References

Allen, G. and Skinner, C. (1991). *Handbook for Research Students in the Social Sciences*. The Falmer Press.

Atkinson, L., Chisholm, V., Dickens, S., Scott, B., Blackwell, J., Tam, F. and Goldberg, S. (1995). Cognitive coping, affective distress and maternal sensitivity: mothers of children with Down's syndrome. *Developmental Psychology*, **31**, 668–676.

Baillie, L. (1995). Ethnography and nursing research: a critical appraisal. *Nurse Researcher*, **3**, 5–21.

Baker, C., Wuest, J. and Stern, P. (1992). Method slurring: the grounded theory/phenomenology example. *Journal of Advanced Nursing*, **17**, 1355–1360.

Barnard, S. (1992). *Delphi study of health care needs of people with disabilities*. Report to Wessex Regional Health Authority.

Beretta, R. (1996). A critical review of the Delphi technique. *Nurse Researcher*, **3**, 79–89.

Bithell, C. (1994). Single subject experimental design: a cause for concern? *Physiotherapy*, **80**, 85–87.

Blanche, E.I. (1995). Alma: coping with culture, poverty and disability. *The American Journal of Occupational Therapy*, **50**, 265–275.

Bond, M. (1995). Progress and procrastination – using a project group to implement changes in service provision for people with disabilities. In *Action Research for Health and Social Care* (E. Hart and M. Bond, eds), pp. 147–162. Open University Press.

Brewer, J. and Hunter, A. (1989). *Multimethod Research: A Synthesis of Styles*. Sage Publications.

Bryman, A. and Burgess, R.G. (1994). *Analyzing Qualitative Data*. Routledge.

Burridge, J., Taylor, P., Hagan, S., Wood, D. and Swain, L. (1997). The effect of common peroneal nerve stimulation on quadriceps spasticity in hemiplegia. *Physiotherapy*, **83**, 82–89.

Cole, P. (1991). How to . . . single subject research designs for clinical and research purposes. *Australian Journal of Physiotherapy*, **37**, 127–128.

Corner, J. (1991). In search of more complete answers to research questions. Quantitative versus qualitative research methods: is there a way forward? *Journal of Advanced Nursing*, **16**, 718–727.

Currier, D.P. (1990). *Elements of Research in Physical Therapy*. Williams and Wilkins.

Dawson, S. and Barker, J. (1995). Hospice and palliative care: a Delphi survey of occupational therapists' roles and training needs. *Australian Occupational Therapy Journal*, **42**, 119–127.

French, S. (1993). *Practical Research: A Guide for Therapists*. Butterworth-Heinemann.

Gill, C., Stratford, P. and Sanford, J. (1992). The use of a single subject design to evaluate a potential adverse effect. *Physiotherapy Canada*, **44**, 25–29.

Glaser, B.G. and Strauss, A.L. (1967). *The Discovery of Grounded Theory: Strategies for Qualitative Research*. Aldine.

Grieve, E. (1993). A fair trial for physiotherapy: the controlled trial. *Physiotherapy*, **79**, 304.

Hartveld, A. and Hegarty, J. (1996). Frequent weight-shift practice with computerised feedback by cerebral palsied children – four single case experiments. *Physiotherapy*, **82**, 573–579.

Hasselkus, B.R. and Dickie, V.A. (1994). Doing occupational therapy: dimensions of satisfaction and dissatisfaction. *American Journal of Occupational Therapy*, **48**, 145–154.

Jones, J. and Hunter, D. (1995). Consensus methods for medical and health services research. *British Medical Journal*, **311**, 376–380.

Larson, E.A. and Fanchiang, S.C. (1996). Life history and narrative research: generating a humanistic knowledge base for occupational therapy. *American Journal of Occupational Therapy*, **50**, 247–249.

Martlew, B. (1996). What do you let the patient tell you? *Physiotherapy*, **82**, 558–565.

McKay, E.A. and Ryan, S. (1995). Clinical reasoning through story telling: examining a student's case story on a fieldwork placement. *British Journal of Occupational Therapy*, **58**, 234–238.

Miles-Tapping, C., Dyck, A., Brunham, S., Simpson, E. and Barber, L. (1990). Canadian therapists' priorities for clinical research: a Delphi study. *Physical Therapy*, **70**, 448–454.

Muecke, M.A. (1994). On the evaluation of ethnographies. In *Critical Issues in Qualitative Research Methods* (J.M. Morse, ed.), pp. 187–209. Sage Publications.

Parry, A. (1991). Physiotherapy and methods of inquiry: conflict and reconciliation. *Physiotherapy*, **77**, 435–438.

Pollock, C., Freemantle, N., Sheldon, T. and Song, F. (1993). Methodological difficulties in rehabilitation research. *Clinical Rehabilitation*, **7**, 63–72.

Protas, E.J., Stanley, R.K., Jankovic, J. and MacNeill, B. (1996). Cardiovascular and metabolic responses to upper and lower extremity exercise in men with idiopathic Parkinson's disease. *Physical Therapy*, **76**, 34–40.

Reynolds, F.A. (1996). Evaluating the impact of an interprofessional communication course through essay content analysis: do physiotherapy and occupational therapy students' essays place similar emphasis on responding skills? *Journal of Interprofessional Care*, **10**, 285–295.

Schmoll, B.J. (1987). Ethnographic inquiry in clinical settings. *Physical Therapy*, **67**, 1895–1897.

Shepard, K.F., Jensen, G.M., Schmoll, B.J., Hack, L.M. and Gwyer, J. (1993). Alternative approaches to research in physical therapy: positivism and phenomenology. *Physical Therapy*, **73**, 88–101.

Sim, J. and Snell, J. (1996). Focus groups in physiotherapy evaluation and research. *Physiotherapy*, 82, 189–198.

Smith, S. (1996). Ethnographic inquiry in physiotherapy research 2. The role of self in qualitative research. *Physiotherapy*, **82**, 349–352.

Stern, P. (1994). Eroding grounded theory. In *Critical Issues in Qualitative Research Methods* (J.M. Morse, ed.), pp. 212–223. Sage Publications.

Stewart, D.W. and Shamdasani, P.N. (1990). *Focus Groups: Theory and Practice*. Sage Publications.

Strauss, A. and Corbin, T. (1990). *Basics of Qualitative Research: Grounded Theory Procedures and Techniques*. Routledge.

Tesch, R. (1990). *Qualitative Research: Analysis Types and Software Tools*. The Falmer Press.

Toomey, M., Nicholson, D. and Carswell, A. (1995). The clinical utility of the Canadian occupational performance measure. *Canadian Journal of Occupational Therapy*, **62**, 242–249.

Townsend, E. (1996). Institutional ethnography: a method for showing how the context shapes practice. *Occupational Therapy Journal of Research*, **16**, 179–199.

Westbrook, M. and McIlwain, D. (1996). Living with the late effects of disability: a five year follow-up survey of coping among post-polio survivors. *Australian Occupational Therapy Journal*, **43**, 60–71.

Complementary reading

Riddoch, J. (1991). Evaluation of practice. *Physiotherapy*, **77**, 439–444.

Robson, C. (1993). *Real World Research: A Resource for Social Scientists and Practitioner-Researchers*. Blackwell. Chapter 6: Designing case studies.

Thomas, J. (1993). *Doing Critical Ethnography*. Sage Publications.

4   Data collection methods: questionnaires

The uses of questionnaires

Questionnaires are popular data collection tools that are widely used in many aspects of our life. For example, most of us will at some point have experienced a market research questionnaire that asks us about our shopping behaviours and preferences. We often have to fill in questionnaires that ask about our social and economic circumstances when applying for government benefits, and around the time of elections, opinion pollsters use responses to questionnaires to try and predict voting behaviour and identify what factors will influence that behaviour. There are many reasons why questionnaires may be used in a health care setting. For example, they may be used to elicit information about patient satisfaction with services or to evaluate patients' responses to treatment. With an increased emphasis on evidence-based practice and customer satisfaction their use is likely to increase in health care settings.

Staples (1991) describes a questionnaire as a standardized list of questions where the order and wording of the questions has been carefully planned. Questionnaires are designed either to be administered by trained interviewers in highly structured face-to-face interviews or as self-administered questionnaires to be completed by respondents when alone or with an interviewer present. In this chapter we will focus on self-administered questionnaires because interviewer-administered questionnaires can be considered as structured interviews which will be covered in Chapter 5.

Types of information that can be elicited from a question

Questions within a questionnaire can be categorized in terms of what kind of information they are trying to elicit. Woodward (1988) states that questions can elicit four different kinds of information. They can extract information about:

1. *Attitudes:* what people say they want.
2. *Beliefs:* what people think is true.
3. *Behaviour:* what people do.
4. *Attributes:* what people are.

While this distinction may seem obvious there is scope for confusion and overlap. For example, Robson (1993) delineated questions into three categories that produce information about facts, behaviours, and beliefs and attitudes. It is not immediately clear how Robson's category of facts relates to any of Woodward's categories. A fact can be defined as a truth or an event that has some permanence. An attribute can be a fact. If you are a woman who was born in England, your attributes are female and English. These attributes cannot be disputed or altered. Behaviours can also be considered to be facts. For example, you may indicate in a market research questionnaire that you always shop at the large supermarket in your town, you use your car to drive to your supermarket and you pay by credit card. Your behaviours are choosing a supermarket, driving to the supermarket and paying for your shopping. While these behaviours cannot be disputed as the truth at the moment when they were reported, they can be influenced or altered. Phipps (1995) used a cross-cultural therapy questionnaire to investigate what factors influenced occupational therapists' work with clients from non-English speaking backgrounds. Issues such as barriers to cross-cultural care were explored as potential influences on occupational therapists' behaviour.

Beliefs and attitudes are slightly more complex. This complexity is partly influenced by a perception that beliefs and attitudes are interrelated; hence Robson's joint category. Yet there is not always agreement as to exactly how they are interrelated. The relationship might be seen as a causal one. For example, your beliefs about the 'supremacy' of men may cause you to have negative attitudes towards women who go out to work. On the other hand, the relationship may simply be correlational. Certain attitudes and beliefs may be linked to one another with no real evidence of a direct causal link. Perhaps in recognition of this complex issue, most research work about attitudes attempts to identify what the attitudes might be and explore influences on those attitudes. For example, Thomson and Lillie (1995) investigated the attitudes of pupils at an integrated and non-integrated school towards children with disabilities. They used the Chedoke–McMaster Attitudes Towards Children with Handicaps scale to compare the attitudes of the two groups of children and assess the influences upon those attitudes.

Ways of eliciting information

While questions can differ in the kinds of information they extract they can also differ in the way that they are stated or presented. Questions can be scaled, open or organizational.

Closed questions

A closed question indicates to the respondent the nature of the response that is expected. Closed questions may be dichotomous, scaled, check-list, grid or ranking in nature. (See Figure 4.1 for examples of scaled questions.)

A dichotomous question forces the respondent to choose between two options (yes/no; OT/PT). Dichotomous questions can cause problems if the options available do not apply to the respondent. For example, the author designed an evaluation questionnaire for a workshop that was run at an Annual Conference of the College of

1. Do you use the university computer workstations to produce written assignments? Please tick appropriate box.

Always	
Sometimes	
Never	

2. Mock biological sciences exams are very useful. Please tick the box that most accurately reflects your level of agreement with this statement.

Strongly agree	Agree	Neither agree nor disagree	Disagree	Strongly disagree

3. Please show, by ticking the appropriate box, which of the faces indicates your overall feeling about your treatment.

☺	
☻	
☹	

Figure 4.1   Examples of scaled questions.

Occupational Therapists. The first question asked people to state whether they were students or clinicians. However, at the workshop there were people who were neither, they were lecturers! Scaled questions provide a scale and ask the respondent to place his/her response somewhere along the scale.

Check-list or multiple choice questions provide a list of responses and ask the respondents to check (tick) one or more of the responses that applies to them.

Examples of multiple choice questions:
1. What were you doing before you started your PT/OT training? Please tick one.
   a) School
   b) Sixth-form college
   c) Full-time access course
   d) Full-time employment
   e) Part-time employment
   f) Housewife/househusband
   g) Unemployed
   h) Other (please specify)

2. What influenced your decision to become an OT or a PT? Please tick more than one answer if appropriate.

> a) Careers advisor suggestion
> b) Relative/friend in the profession
> c) Was a previous OT/PT patient
> d) Pressure from parents
> e) Work experience
> f) Other (please specify)

A grid or matrix question provides the respondent with a matrix. The respondent is expected to fill in each cell in the matrix that is relevant to them (see Figure 4.2).

Ranking questions provide a list of things that the respondents are asked to rank in some way (best to worst, most important to least important).

> **Example of ranking question:**
> 1. Please indicate your level of interest in the course modules listed below. Place a 1 by the module that interests you most, a 2 beside the one you find the next most interesting, and so on.
>   a) Biological sciences
>   b) Group work and ethics
>   c) Teaching and learning
>   d) Discipline-specific modules
>   e) Managing in the workplace
>   f) Behavioural sciences
>   g) Other (please specify)

Open questions

Open questions allow the respondent freedom in the way that they respond. With open questions respondents are not forced to say yes or no, agree or disagree – they are given the scope to say what they think and why. This scope may allow respondents to explain in what circumstances they might answer yes or no, or to outline issues that they feel are important concerning your topic.

What microcomputer(s) do you use with clients?

	TICK IF YOU USE:	PLEASE STATE HOW MANY OF EACH COMPUTER YOU HAVE
BBC computers		
Archimedes computers		
Apple computers		
IBM PCs		

Figure 4.2 Example of a matrix question.

> **Examples of open questions:**
> 1. Please state below your opinions of your clinical supervision during your last clinical fieldwork placement.
> 2. What sources of information did you have available that influenced your decision to purchase/use your current computer? (e.g. equipment brochures, advice from colleagues, advice from IT department.)

Open questions are useful if you want to build on a response to a closed question, if not enough is known to write a closed question or if you want to collect information about a sensitive topic. It is advisable to keep open questions to a minimum unless you can afford to spend a lot of time in analysis.

Organizational questions

In addition to open and closed questions you can include questions in your questionnaire that build on the responses already given or direct the respondent to the right place in the questionnaire. These questions are called funnel and filter questions. A funnel question elicits an initial response and then asks for more and more detail around that response.

> **Example of funnel question:**
> 1. What department do you work in?
> 2. How many staff are there in this department?
> 3. How long have you been working in this department?

Filter questions direct respondents to the next appropriate question that they should answer.

> **Example of filter question:**
> 1. Are you an occupational therapist (OT) or a physiotherapist (PT)?
>   (If you answered OT then go to question 2. If you answered PT go to question 3.)
> 2. What do you think a PT does?
> 3. What do you think an OT does?

Whilst we have highlighted the types of questions that you might include in your questionnaire, others have identified types of questions that you should avoid including in your questionnaire. French (1993), for example, identified five kinds of questions that we should avoid: irrelevant, highbrow, hypothetical, hearsay and kitchen sink questions. Irrelevant questions are those that satisfy curiosity but do not help to answer research question. Highbrow questions are abstract questions with difficult or complicated language. Hypothetical questions ask respondents to imagine what would have happened. They rarely provide useful information and can irritate respondents. Hearsay questions ask one person to give the opinions and attitudes of another, while kitchen sink questions are long and rambling, asking for 'everything but the kitchen sink' (French, 1993, p. 81).

Ensuring a good response rate

We suspect that many people use questionnaires believing that they are an easier option than other data collection methods. Let us put you straight on this! Designing and distributing questionnaires is not an easy option; a lot of hard work needs to be done in order to ensure a good response rate. There are many poorly designed questionnaires distributed that are put straight in the bin and never returned. For a variety of reasons potential questionnaire respondents can become 'disenchanted' (Chesson, 1993, p. 711). Disenchanted respondents and low return rates can be avoided by undertaking several checks, which we will outline in turn.

Check whether a questionnaire is appropriate

A questionnaire might be appropriate if you want to survey large numbers or if the participant population is scattered. If you want to be certain the questions are asked in a standardized manner, then a questionnaire again becomes a logical choice. A questionnaire may be inappropriate, however, if you have small numbers of respondents or if you want to gain in-depth information.

Check the respondent population

It can be useful to briefly outline the characteristics of the research population in order to outline any special needs the respondents may have. Special needs may include things like poor literacy skills, where English is not a first language or failing eyesight. If your research population is mixed and diverse it may be appropriate to use different questionnaires for different subsets, e.g. English and French versions or a small and large print version.

Check the research topic

You need to be clear what your research question is so that you can decide what information you need to ascertain from the questionnaire. You can define your domain (Woodward, 1988) by listing the main topics to be covered. This process enables you to identify topics that are not wholly relevant to your research question, topics which overlap and topics that need to be covered before others are introduced.

Check presentation and layout

Once you have included all the questions you want to ask, it is advisable to check their presentation and layout. You should consider whether your questionnaire is 'user-friendly'. Things that can improve the user-friendly nature of your questionnaire include coloured paper, section titles, sublettered questions, transition statements between sections or questions and allowing adequate space for responses.

Check instructions and information

Potential respondents need information regarding what the research project is about and instructions outlining how they should respond. While this increases the user-friendliness of your questionnaire it also makes it ethical in terms of helping the respondents know exactly what is involved in answering the questionnaire.

Information about the study can be given in the form of a letter or information sheet that can be included with or form part of the questionnaire. The letter or information sheet should state the aim of the study so respondents are fully aware of their involvement and for what purpose the data are being collected. It is not unusual for the covering letter to be left to last and treated as an afterthought. However, given that the letter is the first thing your respondents will see and determines whether they will consent to complete the questionnaire, we should perhaps consider it before anything else. Try to anticipate what questions the respondents would want to ask. Questions might include: What is the study about? Who is conducting the study and where do they come from? What are the benefits for me? How long will it take for me to complete the questionnaire? Will I have to give my name? How do I return the questionnaire?

Try to tailor your information to the target audience and pretest it along with the questionnaire. Ideally, the information should not exceed one page in length, so each sentence will need to be carefully framed and serve a distinct purpose.

Check distribution and follow-up methods

Questionnaires can be distributed by post or by hand. If questionnaires are distributed by hand, then it may be possible for someone to distribute the questionnaires on your behalf. It may improve the response rate if you address the questionnaires to the respondents by name. If you are going to ask respondents to return the questionnaire by a certain date then make sure you don't make them feel rushed. Two weeks is probably the minimum length of time provided the respondent is not under pressure with things like exams, hospital appointments or family illness. Whether or not you follow up people who do not return your questionnaire will depend on practical and ethical issues.

In order to follow someone up for not responding you will need to know who has and has not responded. This usually requires you to precode the questionnaire and make a note of which code goes with which person. By coding the questionnaire you are denying the respondent anonymity. It is fair to say that some people may be put off completing a questionnaire if they see a code of some sort at the top of the questionnaire. They may not want their responses to be traced back to them. Furthermore, codes are there to be cracked and a respondent may spend their time trying to guess what the code means, which is probably not helpful to you or them!

If you do decide to follow up non-respondents then you need to understand that they may not have completed your questionnaire because they were either unable to or did not want to. They may have been unable to complete and return the questionnaire because they had forgotten about the questionnaire, they had lost the questionnaire, they were too busy, they did not have the information the question-naire required or they could not read the questions (literacy and language problems).

Respondents may not want to complete the questionnaire because they do not feel the questionnaire topic is relevant or appropriate, they do not feel the questionnaire is ethical or they do not feel the questionnaire is well presented. By making a decision that they do not want to complete the questionnaire these respondents have withheld consent to take part in your study.

A follow-up is probably going to be effective in targeting those people who have forgotten or lost the questionnaire. Robson (1993) argues that a follow-up letter is probably more effective than a follow-up telephone call in increasing response rates. In the follow-up letter you can emphasize the importance of the study and the value of the respondent's participation. It may be effective to convey surprise and disappointment at non-response, but it is probably not wise to suggest that non-response is common. Make sure you send a further copy of the questionnaire and another stamped addressed envelope. You may need to send as many as three reminders, but Robson (1993:251) warns that reminders are 'subject to the law of diminishing returns'. While you may get frustrated at the small number of returned questionnaires you are receiving, respondents may feel equally frustrated at the constant stream of reminder letters. For each individual respondent there is a point where 'no' really does mean 'no'!

Ensuring useful information is elicited

While we may have done everything we can to ensure a good response to our questionnaire, we also need to ensure that the information we get back is useful. We need to check four main things: the questions, the analysis, accuracy and reliability, and validity.

Checking questions

Irrespective of whether our questions are open or closed we need to check their wording in order to assess whether the respondent can read and respond to them appropriately. Woodward (1988) offers a check-list for assessing the readability of questions. This check-list asks us to consider such issues as the nature of the question (demanding, leading or objectionable) and the meaning of the question (double questions and double negatives). Applying a readability formula can also enable you to check the readability of the overall questionnaire. A readability formula uses counts of language variables in a piece of writing in order to provide an index of probable difficulty for readers (Klare, 1974). For example, Gunning's Fog Index incorporates average sentence length and number of words over three syllables in its calculation:

Reading Grade Level = 0.4 (average sentence length + percentage of words of 3 or more syllables)

The Reading Grade gives some indication of the reading age that would be required of someone to read the text in question. So if a Gunning's Fox Index revealed a Reading Grade Level of 10, that means that someone in Grade 10 at school (14–15 years old) or above would be able to read the text with ease. In the UK, the average reading age of the general population is about 7 years old (Grade 3).

In checking whether respondents can respond to the questions appropriately you need to check the response categories you have provided. The response categories that you give for each question should be sufficient; most people can manage a maximum of seven categories. The categories should also be comprehensive. Make sure you provide a place for every item of information. Allow for all possibilities, but avoid overlap. Your categories should be mutually exclusive categories with only one place on the scale for each item of information.

How respondents answer questions where degree of agreement to a statement has to be indicated can be influenced by a number of factors. Respondents may display a tendency to choose a response category regardless of the question content. They may acquiesce and agree to all statements regardless of their content. Respondents may be influenced by a phenomenon called social desirability, whereby they will not give a response that would be socially unacceptable. The order or position of questions and their response alternatives may also influence respondents. For example, Robson (1993) notes that for questions that require a scaled response, 20% of respondents may use the middle category.

There are several things you can do as a questionnaire designer to reduce these response biases. For acquiescence you can include some checking questions in which you ask the same question but in a different way. For order and positional effects you can change and vary the order in which responses are expected (see Figure 4.3 for examples).

Check the analysis

Useful information is information that you can analyse. Information from a questionnaire may be qualitative or quantitative, descriptive or explanatory. Whatever the nature of the information you will need to find a quick and easy way to organize it so that you can analyse it. This is frequently achieved using a coding system. Codes are symbols, usually numbers, which are used to identify particular responses or types of response (Robson, 1993).

Closed questions are relatively easy to code. The codes can be decided before the questionnaire has been distributed. It can ease analysis to include the codes on the questionnaire (see Figure 4.4 for examples). You can assign any meaning you wish to a coding digit. The code can be arbitrary (e.g. female = 1 and male = 2) or it can be an actual number (e.g. degrees of movement). It is advisable to have a code for non-response; historically this is often 9. This code may be the same or different to codes for don't know, depending on what you want to find out.

For open questions you will need to wait and see what kinds of responses you get before you can start to categorize and code them. Robson (1993) argues that coding of open questions should be based on a substantial, representative sample, selected from the total set of responses. You can copy all the responses to a particular question on to a large sheet of paper matched against the case number given to

Example of checking questions:
1. Physiotherapists should be trained alongside occupational therapists.

Strongly agree	Agree	Neither agree nor disagree	Disagree	Strongly disagree

2. Physiotherapists should not be trained alongside occupational therapists.

Strongly agree	Agree	Neither agree nor disagree	Disagree	Strongly disagree

Example of changing order and position of questions:
1. Physiotherapists should be trained alongside occupational therapists.

Strongly agree	Agree	Neither agree nor disagree	Disagree	Strongly disagree

2. Physiotherapists should be trained alongside nurses.

Strongly disagree	Disagree	Neither agree nor disagree	Agree	Strongly agree

3. Doctors should be trained alongside physiotherapists.

Strongly agree	Agree	Neither agree nor disagree	Disagree	Strongly disagree

4. Chiropractors should be trained alongside physiotherapists.

Strongly disagree	Disagree	Neither agree nor disagree	Agree	Strongly agree

Figure 4.3   Checking for response biases.

Are you an occupational therapist?	CODE
Yes	1
No	2
No response	9

Do you use university computer workstations to produce written assignments?	
Always	1
Sometimes	2
Never	3
No response	9

What were doing before you started your OT/PT training? Please tick one answer.	
School	1
Sixth-form college	2
Full-time access course	3
Full-time employment	4
Part-time employment	5
Housewife/househusband	6
Unemployed	7
Other (please specify)	8
No response	9

Figure 4.4 Examples of codes for closed questions.

each questionnaire. You then need to develop a reasonably small number of categories into which responses can be sorted (see Figure 4.5 for an example).

Question: Please state below your opinions of your clinical supervision during your last clinical fieldwork placement.

Positive comments Code = 1	Negative comments Code = 2
Fun	Intermittent
Thorough	Patronizing
Very helpful	Supervisor never there
Lots of hands-on teaching	Told me off in front of a patient
Watching back assessments was very helpful	What supervision?
Very skilled clinician	Inadequate
Home visit very interesting – good experience	
Broad experience of multi-professional team	
In-service teaching very helpful	

Figure 4.5 Example of coding for open questions.

Check the accuracy

In order to assess whether your questionnaire will provide you with the information you want in the way that you want, it is advisable to pilot or pretest your questionnaire. You can pilot your questionnaire on colleagues or potential respondents. Colleagues may be able to help you gauge how well the questionnaire accomplishes your study objectives. Potential respondents will be able to give feedback on the clarity of instructions and questions and the exhaustiveness of response categories.

In piloting your questionnaire you need to elicit a general impression as well as specific comments on content and wording. Woodward (1988) offers a list of factors to check for in a pilot:

1. Are all the questions understood?
2. Are questions interpreted similarly by all respondents?
3. Do the questionnaire and covering letter create a positive impression?
4. Are the questions answered correctly?

Check the reliability and validity

Reliability and validity will be covered in more detail in Chapter 8. Checking for reliability involves checking for stability and consistency of information. This may involve repeating the same question at several places in the questionnaire or including several questions that ask for the same thing. Checking for validity involves checking for evidence that a questionnaire is collecting information or measuring what it is supposed to measure.

Advantages and disadvantages of questionnaires

Hopefully after reading this chapter you will appreciate that using questionnaires in your research project is not an easy option.

> 'Clearly, questionnaire construction is a complex and time-consuming process and one which should not be entered into lightly. Let the designer be aware!' (Chesson, 1993, p. 713)

The questionnaire designer needs to be aware of the advantages and disadvantages of using questionnaires. Advantages include the fact that questionnaires are relatively cheap to administer, they enable you to gain access to a large number of respondents, there is a low error rate and data from closed questions can be relatively easy to analyse. Disadvantages include the traditional low response rate (40%). If only 40% of the target population return their questionnaires then the representativeness of your sample may be questioned. Questionnaires can also be insensitive to complex issues where a detailed explanation may be necessary in order to make a response understandable. For questionnaires such as patient satisfaction surveys, it may not be appropriate for the questionnaire designer to set the agenda or topics of the questions. Finally, questionnaires may elicit superficial information that requires further probing before the data can be fully understood.

SUPERVISING AND GRADING STUDENTS ON CLINICAL/FIELDWORK PLACEMENT

SECTION ONE: BACKGROUND INFORMATION

1. Name:

2. Address:

3. Are you an OT or a PT?

4. For how many years have you been supervising students (from any school)?

	None		0–5		5+

5. Please indicate by ticking one or more of the options below what the nature of your previous contact with students has been:

Take sole responsibility for supervision	
Supervise jointly with a colleague	
Supervise first years only	
Supervise second years only	
Supervise third years only	
Supervise students at any level	
Supervise one student at a time	
Supervise more than one student at a time	

SECTION TWO: EXPERIENCE OF BRIEFING SESSIONS RUN BY SOUTHSHORE SCHOOL OF OT AND PT

When you attended a briefing session run by Southshore School of Occupational Therapy and Physiotherapy:

6. On a scale of 1 to 10 (10 being extremely useful) how useful did you find the exercise of grading hypothetical students?

7. On a scale of 1 to 10 (1 being extremely easy) how easy did you find it to grade the hypothetical students?

Figure 4.6   Sample questionnaire.

8. In your opinion what do you think you learnt from the briefing exercise?

SECTION THREE: GRADING STUDENTS ON PLACEMENT
9. I found it easy to grade a student from Southshore.

Strongly agree	Agree	Neither agree nor disagree	Disagree	Strongly disagree

10. What were the critical factors for you when trying to grade a Southshore student?

SECTION FOUR: PERSONAL COMMENTS

11. If you would like to make any additional comments about your experience of our briefing sessions and grading Southshore students please feel free to do so in the space below.

Figure 4.6 (*continued*).

EXERCISE

Read the questionnaire in Figure 4.6 entitled 'Supervising and grading students on clinical/fieldwork placement' and answer the following questions:

1. What types of questions (dichotomous, check-list etc.) are questions 3, 4, 5, 8 and 9.
2. Devise a coding scheme for questions 3, 4, 5 and 9.
3. What two questions attempt to check for response consistency?
4. Write an information sheet to accompany this questionnaire.
5. Can you make any suggestions for improving this questionnaire?

Key points

1. Questionnaires can be self-administered or interviewer administered.
2. Questions can elicit information about facts, attitudes, beliefs, behaviours and attributes.
3. Questions can be open, closed or organizational.
4. In order to ensure a good response rate you need to check: appropriateness, respondent population, research topic, presentation, distribution and follow-up.
5. In order to ensure you get useful information you need to check: questions, analysis, accuracy, reliability and validity.
6. There are advantages and disadvantages of using questionnaires.
7. Using questionnaires is not an easy option.

References

Chesson, R. (1993). How to design a questionnaire – a ten stage strategy. *Physiotherapy*, **79**, 711–713.

French, S. (1993). *Practical Research: A Guide for Therapists*. Butterworth-Heinemann.

Klare, G.R. (1974). Assessing readability. *Reading Research Quarterly*, **1**, 62–102.

Robson, C. (1993). *Real World Research. A Resource for Social Scientists and Practitioner-Researchers*. Blackwell.

Phipps, D.J. (1995). Occupational therapy practice with clients from non-English speaking backgrounds: A survey of clinicians in South West Sydney. *Australian Occupational Therapy Journal*, **42**, 151–160.

Staples, D. (1991). Symposium on methodology: questionnaires. *Clinical Rehabilitation*, **5**, 259–264.

Thomson, D.J. and Lillie, L. (1995). The effects of integration on the attitudes of non-disabled pupils to their disabled peers. *Physiotherapy*, **81**, 746–752.

Walker, E.M. (1996). Questionnaire design in practice. *British Journal of Therapy and Rehabilitation*, **3**, 229–233.

Woodward, C.A. (1988). Questionnaire construction and question writing for research in medical education. *Medical Education*, **22**, 347–363.

Complementary reading

Bell, J. (1987). *Doing Your Research Project*. Open University Press.

Del Greco, L. and Walop, W. (1987). Questionnaire development: 1. Formulation. *CMAJ*, **136**, 583–585.

Del Greco, L. and Walop, W. (1987). Questionnaire development: 5. The pre-test. *CMAJ*, **136**, 1025–1026.

Del Greco, L., Walop, W. and Eastridge, L. (1987). Questionnaire development: 3. Translation. *CMAJ*, **136**, 817–818.

Del Greco, L., Walop, W. and McCarthy, R.H. (1987). Questionnaire development: 2. Validity and reliability. *CMAJ*, **136**, 699–700.

Walop, W., Del Greco, L., Eastridge, L., Marchand, B. and Szentveri, K. (1987). Questionnaire development: 4. Preparation for analysis. *CMAJ*, **136**, 927–928.

5 Data collection methods: interviews

Why interview?

'An interview is a kind of conversation; a conversation with a purpose . . . a flexible and adaptable way of finding things out.' (Robson, 1993, p. 228)

Interviews are means of getting rich descriptive information from people who have experienced the event you wish to investigate in your research. They are commonly used in social research and are increasingly being used to add depth and colour to the more traditional quantitative medical research. Of course, interviewing patients comes as second nature to therapists and using interviews to gather research data may seem at first glance to be an easy option. But Britten (1995, p. 311) warns against assuming this, stating that when interviewing patients '. . . the clinical task is to fit that problem into an appropriate medical category' whilst 'in a qualitative research interview the aim is to discover the interviewee's own framework of meanings'. French (1993) too suggests that therapists may have slipped into bad interviewing techniques over their years of practice and these may need to be unlearned before research interviews can take place.

Interviews are very useful for finding out about people's behaviour, experiences, opinions, beliefs, feelings, knowledge and background (Patton, 1990). An interview allows you to talk to your subject and elicit more information than is possible from a questionnaire. Face-to-face interviews also allow you to observe non-verbal communication and, if held in the person's home or place of work, their interaction with their environment. An interview allows you to pick up points of interest and delve more deeply.

Interviews will give different information from an alternative perspective to that of quantitative research. A quantitative project looking at the outcome of occupational therapy stress management classes in a community mental health setting will give you useful information about changes in prescribed drug use, return to work and number of relapses. Interviewing the participants and therapists, however, will give much more descriptive information about the impact of the sessions on the actual lives of the participants. In many cases it is appropriate to collect both numerical data and conduct qualitative interviews in a research project, as this gives a rounded evaluation of a service or intervention, although some authors warn that the differences in approach may confound rather than clarify (Bryman, 1992).

THERAPY EXAMPLE

Cullen-Erikson (1994) used interviews to gain useful information about the achievement of an activity of daily living skill by children with learning disabilities. Cullen-Erikson wanted to explore the area of daily dental hygiene from the perspective of the parents of children with learning disabilities. She felt that, although there was a considerable amount of questionnaire data already available, the information had not provided 'the background context for behaviours and opinions, or discovered the subtle nuances in the culture studied'. She also found that in other studies where interviews had been conducted 'information of a greater depth was obtained'. Six interviews were undertaken with parents of children with learning disabilities that identified four key themes. Cullen-Erikson felt that, although the size and design of the project limited its generalizability, 'it has provided some new insights into an area that has received too little attention to date'.

Interview lengths vary between several minutes and an hour and a half. The style and length of the interview will vary according to the information you seek. During this period the researcher asks questions or asks the interviewee to comment on statements.

EXERCISE

Think about the last time you spoke with a friend or colleague for about an hour then jot down all the topics you covered. Write down as much of the factual detail that you can remember from this conversation, then the opinions, feelings and beliefs that were expressed. Perhaps there were some strong emotions too. See if you can remember some actual quotes spoken during that conversation. Note the environment where this conversation took place, any things that you or your friend said that may have been influenced by the environment and any bits of the conversation where you think your friend's body language or tone of voice did not seem to match up with the words he or she spoke. Now jot down what you remember as being the three key points. Ask the person you had the conversation with to do the same and compare notes. Think about how much of that information you could have got by presenting your friend with a list of questions on the topics you discussed. Finally, have a think about whether the conversation would have been the same if you had talked about the same subjects with someone else. Would any common themes have emerged even if the points of view were different?

This exercise will give you some idea of the breadth of subjects it is possible to cover in one short hour or the depth you can achieve just discussing one topic. It will also give you an idea of how much information is going to be collected from an interview and how difficult it can be to remember all the minutiae of the conversation, including memorable quotes. It may also show the influence of the environment where the conversation took place and the importance of noting the tone of voice and body language as well as actual words spoken. You may be surprised that your perception of the key points of the conversation can differ to that of the other participant. Would you have got this depth of data from a questionnaire? Would that have mattered? If you were simply talking about the price of supermarket shopping, a questionnaire would have sufficed; but if you wanted to understand the frustrations associated with queuing, parking and out of town shopping, then it would have been very much more difficult to ascertain the breadth of true feelings without having had a conversation. This exercise emphasizes several points to remember when deciding whether to conduct interviews:

1. An interview will generate a terrific amount of data that then have to be analysed.
2. Do you need this wealth of data or will a questionnaire suffice?
3. An interview will allow you to probe for more information relevant to the initial response.
4. Unless you record your interview in some way at the time or immediately afterwards you will lose a lot of data or your memory may skew the actual responses or emotions behind those responses.
5. The environment in which an interview takes place may influence the interview.
6. It is important to match the words someone says to their body language or tone of voice.
7. It is important to check the content of your interview data with the participant to ensure that your perception is the same as theirs (validity).

One of the reasons why 'hard' scientists can view interview data with suspicion is because it is impossible to obtain true reliability between interviews. In a semi-structured or unstructured interview each interviewee may lead you down different paths, making it difficult to match responses. However, this very anomaly ensures the validity of the interview, i.e. the interviewee is able to express their true feelings about elements of the topic that have meaning for them. Reliability is easier to obtain in a structured interview where questions are formalized, i.e. asked in exactly the same way and in the same order for each interviewee. However, even here there can be issues of inter-rater reliability. One interviewer could ask the question 'How do *you* feel about that?' while another interviewer could ask 'How do you *feel* about that?', and both would obtain different answers from differing perspectives. More information on the reliability and validity of interviews can be found in Chapter 11 and Barriball and While (1994).

It is almost inevitable that you will approach your research with some kind of bias. Quantitative research accounts for this by identifying a one-tailed hypothesis which may predict not only that an intervention will have an effect, but also what that effect will be. The onus on the quantitative researcher is to show that this effect does indeed occur and that it is probable that this effect did not happen by chance. The qualitative nature of research based on semi-structured or unstructured interviews is not hypothesis driven and, in theory, should allow all aspects of the experience under investigation to be researched, however bizarre or unexpected the outcome. In practice this is very difficult. For example, a therapist seeking to explore the experiences of children with disabilities may have strong personal feelings about the education and rehabilitation of children which must impact the research, both in the questions asked at interview and the analysis. DePoy and Gitlin (1993, p. 277) state that:

> 'Although investigator bias cannot be eliminated, it can be identified and examined in terms of its impact on data collection processes and interpretive accounts'.

This process of self-examination is known as reflexivity. The researcher needs to reflect not only on their perspective of the topic but also on why they hold that view and how they come to hold it. Our therapy researcher in the above example needs to write down his/her personal views about the education and rehabilitation of children with disabilities and decide why they hold these views, what led to them, how they have been reinforced and why they are important. It is important to acknowledge the strength of these views and whether they come from any particular perspective, e.g. a political stance or specific social class. It is useful to write this reflection in your personal project journal (see Chapter 13) and revisit it from time to time to keep a check on the gathering and interpretation of data. It may be important to your research to highlight researcher bias and the methods employed to account for this.

Types of interview

There are five main types of interview: structured, semi-structured, unstructured, focus groups and telephone.

Structured interviews

Structured interviews are just that; highly formalized often having precoded responses. This is a format commonly used by market researchers. Questions are read from a sheet and always in the same order to each interviewee. The answers are already fixed and the interviewee simply has to choose the one most pertinent to his or her views. The interviewer tries to ensure reliability by asking each question in the same way with the same voice inflection. This sort of interview seeks to obtain factual answers rather than richness of opinion (see Figure 5.1 for an example). Structured interviews are considered to be reliable and quick, the interviewer having maximum control (Smith, 1995). The sort of questions that are asked include:

1. Dichotomous questions ('yes/no' or 'employed/unemployed').
2. Multiple choice questions ('Which of these five chocolate bars is your favourite?').
3. Scaled questions ('Would you describe your health as excellent, good, fair or poor?').

> 1. How long have you worked in this burns unit? <1 year, 1–3 years, >3 years
> 2. What grade are you?   junior, senior 2, senior 1, supt, other
> 3. How many beds in the unit?   (count)
> 4. Do you have open referral to physiotherapy?   yes/no
> 5. How stressful do you find this work?   not at all/quite/very/extremely
> 6. Would you say you cope with the death of young patients with burns:
>   very well, quite well, badly, extremely badly?
> 7. Do you have the opportunity to discuss the effect that working on the
>   burns unit may have on you with anyone?   yes/no
> 8. If yes, is this opportunity (*show card to enable participant to choose response*):
>   formal – set up by employers; informal – *ad hoc* peer support; informal –
>   from friends and family away from work; formal – privately arranged
>   counselling?

Figure 5.1   Part of a hypothetical structured interview investigating the impact of working in a burns unit on the role of the physiotherapist.

Occasionally there is room at the end of a structured interview for more descriptive information, for example 'Do you have any other comments to make about your stay in hospital?'. However, this type of interview does not account for any exploration of that question, it simply allows the analysis to pick up recurring points that were not adequately addressed in the main questionnaire.

Administering a structured interview takes less time than other types of interviews. It also allows easy statistical analysis of the gathered data, as responses are already predetermined and easily coded. If your structured interview comprises multiple choice questions it is a good idea to carry cards with the choice of answers on them to show to interviewees rather than hope they can remember all the choices you read out. There may seem to be very little difference between a structured interview and a questionnaire and indeed this is true. One advantage to using a structured interview over a questionnaire is that the participants will not see it, so it is not so important to make it attractive. Similarly, the interviewer is present to clarify if there is any misunderstanding of questions (Drummond, 1996). The response rate for questionnaires can be around 40% but this rises considerably when you make an appointment for an interview (Bowling, 1997). The disadvantages include the interviewee not believing that their responses will be anonymous despite assurances and the researcher time involved in interviewing compared with putting postal questionnaires into envelopes (Drummond, 1996). Weller (1988) considers structured interviewing in more depth.

Semi-structured interviews

These are much less formal than structured interviews and work to an interview schedule rather than a spoken list of questions. These interviews are far more interactive, with the interviewer using communication techniques akin to counselling skills to ascertain information (French, 1993). Remember, however, that you are conducting an interview and be careful not to fall into the counselling role. The interviewer draws up the schedule based on topics, questions and prompts. It is not necessary to follow the order of these; the schedule is there simply to ensure that the interviewer covers all the areas under investigation, to keep the interview on track and to act as a prompt if the interviewee dries up.

Returning to our hypothetical project investigating the impact of working in a burns unit on the role of physiotherapists, we might

---

Topic 1. Role of the physiotherapist in the burns unit.
Question: How long have you worked here?
Prompts: length of time
            ? rotational post
            ? specializing in this field

Question: What do you do here in a typical day?
Prompts: structure of day
            ward rounds/meetings
            teaching/in-service training
            treating patients
            emergencies/on-calls

Question: What are the differences between working on a burns unit and a general ward?
Prompts: daily routine
            work-load
            relationships with staff
            relationships with patients/relationships with relatives

Topic 2. Impact of this setting on the physiotherapist
Question: How does working on a burns unit affect you?
Prompts: professionally (work experience, staff team)
            physically (? more tired, heat)
            emotionally (?exciting, upsetting, standing back)
            mentally (?stimulating, affecting sleep/relationships, depressing)

Question: Describe an incident in the burns unit that made an impact on you?
Prompts: professional
            patient/relative
            staff/multi-disciplinary team

Question: What sort of situation at work might prompt you to seek support?
Prompts: death of patient
            children with burns
            distressed patients/relatives/staff
            professional issues (staffing levels/time/resources)

Question: Where can you go for support if you are feeling . . . (as interviewee describes above)?
Prompts: counselling/pastoral care/management support at work
            peer support
            family/friends

Question: What sort of impact has working in the burns unit had on you?
Prompts: as a person
            as a physiotherapist

Figure 5.2 Hypothetical interview schedule for a project investigating the impact of working in a burns unit.

decide we want to explore two key topics, the role of the physiotherapist in the burns unit and the impact of this setting on the
physiotherapist. Under these two headings we develop questions.
These will be open-ended questions that are designed to stimulate
responses in the topic area. A semi-structured interview also contains
prompts to remind the interviewer to draw out more specific
information. These are often in the form of bullet points, as they are
an *aide-mémoire* for the interviewer to use as appropriate with each
interviewee, not formal questions. Start with general questions that are
non-threatening and which are easy to answer. Some of these
questions might necessarily be closed (e.g. 'how long have you worked
here?') but go some way to putting the interviewee at ease, especially
if your later questions are going to be searching. See Figure 5.2 for a
hypothetical interview schedule for a project investigating the impact
of working in a burns unit on the role of the physiotherapist.

Unstructured interviews

Unstructured interviews allow the interviewee to take control, with
the interviewer prompting them to explore the issues and opinions
they raise in more depth. They are commonplace in psychiatry and
psychology and may well allow people's true feelings and views to
emerge (Robson, 1993) unfettered by the restraints of an interviewer's
agenda. Although this allows the participant to identify the issues that
are pertinent to them, there is always the danger that they can get
carried away and lead right away from the original topic. Although
this may be what the interviewer wants in some cases, they are more
likely to want the interviewee to stay within some boundaries, so it is
perfectly allowable to focus the interview. By focusing the unstructured interview the interviewer is able to ascertain information
about a topic that is completely from the interviewee's perspective but
is still able to analyse the data relative to the initial research topic. An
interview guide with a broad topic area and flexible parameters, rather
than a schedule, helps to keep the interview on track (see Figure 5.3
for an example). Unstructured interviews, moreso than the other types,
require a degree of articulation on the part of the interviewee (French,
1993).

Focus groups

Focus groups are a type of group interview, comprising eight to
twelve individuals who all have something in common, that is, an

---

Tell me what it is like to be a physiotherapist on the burns unit.
[Keep within the following parameters:

physiotherapy
burns unit
experiences of working in burns unit
impact of working in burns unit on self as individual/therapist]

Figure 5.3   A hypothetical interview guide for a project investigating the impact
of working in a burns unit on the role of the physiotherapist.

opinion on the topic being investigated. A facilitator, often one of the researchers, leads the group discussion along the same lines as a semi-structured or unstructured interview. Another researcher is usually present to record any pertinent observations such as non-verbal behaviour for use in the subsequent analysis. The interactions between the group members and the way in which they approach and explore different aspects of the topic under discussion can give valuable insight into opinions about that topic. It is important to stress that focus groups do not seek to reach a consensus, rather a range of points of view around the topic area.

> 'The focus group technique is especially well suited for problems in health research where complex clinical issues are often best explored through a qualitative approach'. (Carey, 1994, p. 227)

Topics suitable for investigation through focus groups might include therapists' perceptions of continuing professional development, or clients' and carers' views of services provided by a community learning disability team. More information about conducting focus groups can be found in Carey (1994), Bowling (1997) and Stewart and Shamdasani (1990).

Telephone interviews

Telephone interviewing is an attractive alternative to face-to-face interviewing, saving time and money on travel. It is also safer for the interviewer, who can interview from the comfort of their own office and for the interviewee who may be apprehensive about meeting a stranger. Information may be gathered quickly and over a wide geographical area, enabling large numbers of people to be contacted. Drummond (1996) notes the potential for gathering accurate data about activities of daily living from telephone interviews with past patients. However, she warns against possible bias in sampling as, although the majority of people now have telephones, it could be easy to exclude people who have answer-phones or who are not available during the normal working day. Bowling (1997) found the number of call-backs required to 'catch' some subjects very time-consuming. Other considerations are the cost of the calls and the fact that some people will be automatically excluded, e.g. deaf people and some people with learning disabilities. Telephone interviews may be conducted in any of the interviewing styles: structured, semi-structured or unstructured, although structured interview style surveys are the most common. Agreement to be interviewed is greater if the interviewee is forewarned in an information and request letter and possibly given an appointment time for the call. Sensitivity is required on the part of the interviewer to ensure that the interviewee is not irritated by a call in the middle of meal-times or too late in the evening. Another variable that cannot be accounted for by the researcher is the presence of distractions such as children or boiling pots at the interviewee's end. People considering interviewing by telephone are advised to read Groves et al. (1998) and Drummond (1996) for further information.

Collecting interview data

Once you have your interviewee talking it is necessary to record their responses for later analysis. A structured questionnaire takes care of itself, as you simply record the respondent's choice of answer to each question. Questions asked in a telephone survey can be similarly recorded. Recording a semi-structured or unstructured interview or focus group is more complicated. Note taking during the interview is a recognized method of recording, although some researchers feel that this impinges on the flow of the interview. An alternative is to write down notes as soon as possible after the interview.

Tape recording is a useful alternative. The advantages of tape recording are that the flow of the interview is not interrupted by note taking and the entire conversation can be replayed and transcribed for detailed analysis. Disadvantages include anxiety of the interviewee leading to the situation where your most valuable information comes after the tape has been turned off at the end of the interview. It is essential for the researcher to be confident with tape recording through lots of practice prior to the actual interviewing. Check that your microphone will record adequately in the interview setting and ensure you have enough tapes and batteries. Remember that a standard C90 tape will run out after three-quarters of an hour, which can be a bit difficult when your interview lasts an hour, especially when your best information often comes at around this time when the interviewee has relaxed and warmed to the topic. It may be better to change tapes where there is a natural break earlier on in the interview. This will also help with transcription (see Chapter 11). It is also possible to record telephone interviews, although it is very important that the interviewees know they are being recorded and consent to that.

Before you decide on which recording method to use think about how you are going to analyse the information (see also Chapters 9 and 11). If you require quotes to add the personal insights of participants it is better to tape record so that accurate quotes may be obtained and put into the context in which they were said. However, it can take between six and ten hours to transcribe a taped one-hour interview. This time increases if there are many voices on the tape such as from a focus group. Unless you can afford some secretarial time it is you who will have to transcribe prior to analysing the data (see Chapters 11 and 16).

In order to achieve some consistency between interviews it is important that the style of interview does not vary either between interviews or between interviewers. Some reliability between interviews can be obtained by interviewing in the same or similar surroundings. For example, if you are interviewing therapists, you may choose to interview them all in their departments after work rather than one in the department, another in their own home and another in your office. Where more than one interviewer is undertaking the research, training is important to achieve consistency (Bowling, 1997).

Interviewing skills

Good questions in research interviewing should be open ended, neutral, sensitive and clear to the interviewee (Patton, 1980). Robson (1993) highlighted four main skills for conducting research interviews:

1. Listen more than you speak!
2. Put your questions in a straightforward, clear and non-threatening way.
3. Avoid giving cues that might influence the response, for example asking leading questions such as 'You enjoy your work, don't you?' or 'Would you agree that you are working towards evidence-based practice?'. Some interviewees will answer to please the interviewer rather than give their own opinion.
4. Enjoy the experience! Try not to look tired, bored or scared; remember interviewees quickly pick up your non-verbal communication and they will react accordingly.

Examples of these skills include those that facilitate the flow of the interview and encourage the participant to open up. Counselling techniques including empathy, reflection of meaning, reflection of feeling and summarizing can all be employed in semi-structured and unstructured interviewing (Egan, 1994). An ability to establish a good rapport with a wide range of people (Bowling, 1997) and sensitivity, knowing when to delve and when to pull back, are also useful skills.

Bad questions are those that are:

1. Ambiguous: 'How long have you been here?'
2. Vague: 'What are patients like?'
3. Double barrelled: 'Do you like working here or was your last job better?'
4. Contain jargon: 'Did you have CPM immediately after your knee arthroplasty?'
5. Leading: 'List the benefits you got from attending the stroke group.'
6. Biased: 'Did you benefit more from daily outpatient treatment than from a monthly domicillary visit?'
7. Aggressive: 'I'll ask you again. Which treatment caused you the most pain?'

Conducting interviews in practice

The following process is a useful guide to conducting interviews in practice.

1. Research the background to your topic area.
2. Decide what type of interview would best suit your methodology, topic and subject cohort.
3. Design your interview questions/schedule/guide.
4. Pilot your interview content, technique, style, competency with note taking or tape recording.
5. Gain permission to access your subject cohort if appropriate (see Chapter 17).
6. Send information letters to potential participants.
7. Make appointments to interview participants. Be considerate of

their needs. Do not take clinicians away from patient time. Remember that disabled interviewees may be put under a lot of stress to be ready for an early morning appointment. Similarly, both interviewer and interviewee may be too tired to conduct a useful interview after a long day at work.

8. Arrange to hold the interview in a room where you will not be interrupted – preferably one without a telephone. If possible, ensure mobile phones and bleeps are switched off for the duration of the interview. The venue should be quiet and without distraction. Ensure that it is not possible for others to overhear the interview, as this would compromise confidentiality.

9. Turn up on time!

10. Dress appropriately: 'power dressing' may inhibit teenage interviewees and children; older people may not take you seriously if you arrive wearing torn jeans and nose rings; wearing uniform may inhibit some people but put others at ease (French, 1993).

11. Arrange the room so that it is conducive to easy conversation. Placing chairs at right angles (or in a circle for a focus group) rather than directly opposite each other or on either side of a desk reduces formality. Place any microphone so that it is unobtrusive but able to pick up the voices of all participants.

12. Welcome the interviewee and introduce yourself and them to each other in a focus group. Focus groups usually comprise participants who have never met before, so facilitators often break the ice with refreshments prior to the actual group.

13. Explain the purpose of the research and the interview.

14. Explain the content, style and length of the interview.

15. Ask interviewees to sign an informed consent form. Some ethics committees require researchers to obtain two signatures: one consenting to be interviewed, the other consenting to being tape recorded.

16. Conduct the interview, starting with some general, non-intrusive questions to put the interviewee at ease and allow the interviewer to get into their stride.

17. Close the interview within the stated time, thanking the interviewee.

18. If you want the interviewee to validate the transcript or your analysis ask them before they leave, giving details of when you will be sending the paperwork and when you require their response.

19. Immediately after the interview make any notes necessary for your later analysis.

20. Some interviewees will be interested in the results of your project. Remember to send an abstract or summary to individual interviewees or the person who was key in obtaining their co-operation, e.g. therapy manager or chair of self-help group.

Searching for meaning

Interviews in research must be used to address the research question. Looking back at the three hypothetical interviews in this chapter it is interesting to see if they address adequately the research question, namely 'What is the impact of working in a burns unit on the role of the physiotherapist?'. The interview questions of the structured interview make the assumption that physiotherapists working in burns units will be affected by the stressful nature of the job and may need to use support services. The researcher may have devised the question list based on this assumption or they may have constructed the questions after observing physiotherapists working in this situation. Either way it only allows the researcher to investigate one particular aspect of the work. This may seem rather restrictive, but if the questions originate from a specific research question relating to the impact of treating patients in stressful situations then this is entirely valid. However, if the interviewee feels that the stress they experience in their job is related more to, say, relationships within the multi-disciplinary team, then there is no scope for exploring this in this structured interview.

As previously indicated, the structured interview allows the interviewee to choose a reply which 'pigeon-holes' responses, not allowing for any flexibility. For example, in question 5 'How stressful do you find this work?' the real response of the interviewee may be 'It depends. When the unit is full it is very stressful but when we are not so busy I do not feel any stress at all'. Which response most closely matches this answer? Careful piloting of structured interview questions will highlight such anomalies and allow for correction. Once you are sure your structured interview question list is watertight you will benefit from being able to collect data quickly and will reap the benefits of easily codable responses when you come to analyse the data.

By allowing you to delve more deeply into feelings and opinions, semi-structured interviews do not suffer from the same problems of deciding which answer most closely reflects the interviewee's response. However, you can see from the interview schedule that the interviewer is still being fairly directive in their questioning. The unstructured interview allows the interviewee free range of expression. Note the parameters in the hypothetical example. There is no mention of stress or coping strategies and, although the researcher may hypothesize that this area is key, the unstructured interview allows the physiotherapist being interviewed to discuss any topics of importance to him or her about working on a burns unit. Often informal, unstructured interviews can inform the schedule of a subsequent semi-structured or structured interview.

Examples of interviews from the literature

Broom and Williams (1996) investigated occupational stress amongst neurological rehabilitation physiotherapists. Individual semi-structured interviews were undertaken by a single researcher with ten physiotherapists of mixed grades to ascertain levels and impact of occupational stress. Permission was obtained from the physiotherapy superintendents prior to sending copies of the research protocol to prospective interviewees for information. The interviewer was herself a physiotherapist, which she feels was an advantage, allowing her to both gain access and collect high quality data. Also, '. . . she was perceived as having an understanding of the physiotherapists' work, yet posing no threat to their jobs or status'. The interviews were recorded and transcribed in full: 'a process which helped strengthen the validity of the data by avoiding selective recording of information'. Four key areas were identified from the transcribed data. The researchers refer to previous research in the discussion of their findings, opening further debate in this area.

Harrison and Barlow (1995) attempted to obtain a consumer perspective on outpatient therapeutic services. The researchers sought to obtain patients' views on the quality of therapeutic outpatient services. It was felt to be important that patients were allowed more freedom to explore their views than a predetermined questionnaire survey would allow. They chose to hold a focus group, inviting six patients by prior arrangement to a quiet area in the physiotherapy department. Participants were offered a drink and the procedure of the group was explained. They were invited to make some personal notes about the topic area before the discussion was facilitated 'in a non-directive, conducive manner'. Notes were taken during the discussion, which were read back to participants at the end 'for verification, amendment and prioritization'. The researchers felt that this method allowed the patients' perspective to be identified and added to the views of clinicians and providers, which 'may thus provide a more balanced view of services'.

Booth and Booth (1996) conducted narrative research with 'inarticulate' subjects. The researchers wished to explore the viability of identifying the views, experiences and opinions of people with learning disabilities through narrative research. They identified inarticulateness, unresponsiveness and problems with time as being some of the inhibitors to obtaining information from this client group. In a single case study the researchers explored the experience of gaining narrative from one man through various interviewing techniques. They felt that, despite the time involved and the difficulties in obtaining 'good text', the research produced useful data, concluding that 'the emphasis of research should be on overcoming the barriers that impede the involvement of inarticulate subjects instead of highlighting the difficulties they present'.

Key points

1. Interviews offer the opportunity to obtain rich descriptive data. The researcher needs to identify his/her perspective on the research topic in order to account for any potential bias.
2. Interviews may take different forms including structured, semi-structured, unstructured, telephone interviews and focus groups.
3. Interview data must be collected with a view to their analysis. Interviews may be tape recorded or notes should be made during or immediately after the interview.

4. Interviewing skills, including clear delivery of questions and appropriate demeanour of the interviewer, are key to obtaining good data. Bad questions can lead to ambiguity and biased data.

5. In practice the research topic needs to be researched by the interviewer to ensure appropriate questions are raised. The venue, organization and process of the interview are important. Interviewees may appreciate a summary of the results of the research.

References

Barriball, K.L. and While, A. (1994). Collecting data using a semi-structured interview: a discussion paper. *Journal of Advanced Nursing*, **19**, 328–335.

Booth, T. and Booth, W. (1996). Sounds of Silence: narrative research with inarticulate subjects. *Disability and Society*, **11**, 55–69.

Bowling, A. (1997). *Research Methods in Health: Investigating Health and Health Services*. Open University Press.

Britten, N. (1995). Qualitative interviews in medical research. *British Medical Journal*, **311**, 251–253.

Broom, J.P. and Williams, J. (1996). Occupational stress and neurological rehabilitation. *Physiotherapy*, **82**, 606–613.

Bryman, A. (1992). *Quantity and Quality in Social Research*. Routledge.

Carey, M.A. (1994). The group effect in focus groups: planning, implementing and interpreting focus group research. In *Critical Issues in Qualitative Research Methods*. (J.M. Morse, ed.), pp. 225–241. Sage Publications.

Cullen-Erikson, M. (1994). Parent's experiences in assisting a person with an intellectual disability to achieve optimal dental health. *Australian Occupational Therapy Journal*, **41**, 163–172.

DePoy, E. and Gitlin, L.N. (1993). *Introduction to Research: Multiple Strategies for Health and Human Services*. Mosby.

Drummond, A. (1996). *Research Methods for Therapists*. Chapman & Hall.

Egan, G. (1994). *The Skilled Helper: A Problem-Management Approach to Helping*. Brooks/Cole Publishing Company.

French, S. (1993). *Practical Research: A Guide for Therapists*. Butterworth-Heinemann.

Groves, R.M., Biemer, P.P., Lyberg, L.E., Massey, J.T., Nicholls, W.L. and Waksberg, J. (1988). *Telephone Survey Methodology*. John Wiley.

Harrison, K. and Barlow, J. (1995). Focus group technique: a consumer perspective on outpatient therapeutic services. *British Journal of Therapy and Rehabilitation*, **2**, 323–327.

Patton, M.Q. (1990). *Qualitative Evaluation and Research Methods*. Sage Publications.

Robson, C. (1993). *Real World Research: A Resource for Social Scientists and Practitioner-Researchers*. Blackwell.

Smith, J. (1995). Semi-structured interviewing and qualitative analysis. In *Rethinking Methods in Psychology*. (J.A. Smith., R. Harre and L. Van Langenhove, eds), pp. 9–26. Sage Publications.

Stewart, D.W. and Shamdasani, P.N. (1990). *Focus Groups: Theory and Practice*. Sage Publications.

Weller, S. (1988). *Systematic Data Collection*. Sage Publications.

Complementary reading

Holstein, J.A. and Gubrium, J.F.(1995) *The Active Interview*. Sage Publications.

McCracken, G. (1988). *The Long Interview*. Sage Publications.

6　Data collection methods: observation

The use of observation

Observation is possibly an underused data collection method in therapy research, yet in some ways it may be the most natural method to use.

> 'Observation is in some ways rather like breathing: life depends on it and we do it all the time'. (Peberdy, 1993, p. 47)

Observation is a skill that all therapists employ in their daily work. In making assessments and planning treatment programmes clinicians rely heavily on watching their patients' behaviour. They are skilled observers and these skills can be used in research. Observation may also provide additional information that other methods of data collection are unable to obtain. For example, Black (1996) argues that observation can place interventions used in randomized controlled trials in a context of patient and clinician beliefs, wishes and attitudes.

An observer can gain research data from what they see and what they hear. They may see and hear as an 'outsider' or as an 'insider', being separate from or part of the situation under observation. Observation can be used to study the behaviour of people as well as the situation in which that behaviour takes place. In addition to watching and listening, observation may involve talking and reading. It can be acceptable to interview those being observed or to read documents obtained from the observation site. Observation can be used as a data collection tool on its own or as part of an assortment of data collection tools. Observation can be used in qualitative and quantitative research and can offer researchers useful information as part of a main research project or as part of a pilot or exploratory study.

Structured and unstructured observation

Observations can differ in terms of how structured they are. They can be structured, semi-structured or unstructured. Structured observations attempt to categorize information in a particular and methodical way. Behaviours to be observed are defined and put into categories. The observer knows what they are looking for prior to the observation periods. Structured observation can be achieved in natural and manipulated environments.

In unstructured observation there is no attempt to define or predict what will be observed before the observation session. Observers go into unstructured observation prepared to observe anything and everything. In unstructured observations researchers are usually trying to capture the whole picture. They are interested in the total situation rather than specific, individual aspects of it. In additional to being whole, the picture has to be as natural as possible with little disturbance or manipulation. In unstructured observations information is commonly recorded through the use of field notes. Field notes can be written during or after the observation sessions. They are commonly conceptualized as an 'observer's diary'.

Observers who engage in semi-structured observations will have some idea of what they wish to observe but allow themselves the flexibility to record any extraordinary or unexpected events that may occur during an observation session.

Data analysis can also vary depending on the type of observation that is being conducted. Analysis can take place during an observation session or afterwards. With semi-structured and unstructured observation, analysis commonly occurs while the observer is observing. This allows the observer an opportunity to adapt and change what and how they observe depending on what the results indicate and highlight.

Structured, unstructured and semi-structured observations can be employed in a single observation session or at different times and stages of an observation project. An observer needs to be clear what their research purpose and question is before deciding how structured or unstructured their observations should be.

Structured and unstructured observations have their advantages and disadvantages. In unstructured observation researchers are often having to make inferences as to why something happened or the significance of an occurrence. Making inferences like this can be considered to be subjective and opens the research up to claims of poor reliability and validity. However, the information obtained from unstructured observation is often argued to be 'richer' than that obtained from a more structured approach. What 'richer' means may be open to many interpretations. It may mean more interesting, more in depth or more relevant. Generally, if the data is richer then it may actually mean that it is more valid because it is providing a more authentic description or measurement. Pretzlik (1994) offers a comparison of structured and unstructured observations which highlights other practical advantages and disadvantages (see Table 6.1).

Participant and non-participant observation

A distinction is often made between four observation roles. These roles can be put at different places on a spectrum in terms of how involved the researcher is in the groups they are observing (Robson, 1993; French, 1993; Peberdy, 1993). The four roles are complete participant, participant as observer, observer as participant and complete observer. The complete participant acts as a full and ordinary member of the group, while the complete observer has no contact with the group at all. An example of a study that falls in between these two extremes of observation is that of Smith (1996). In an observational study of

Table 6.1 Advantages and disadvantages of structured and unstructured observation

	Advantages	Disadvantages
Structured	Suitable for large-scale studies. Can provide measurable, quantifiable data. Useful for testing hypotheses. Strong reliability. Easy to train observers. Cost and time effective.	Predetermined categories can neglect essential information. Can provide only a partial description of the whole situation. The context in which the data are collected is largely ignored.
Unstructured	Considers complexity of the situation. Little equipment is necessary. Little preparation is needed. Allows a more creative way of looking at the world.	Time-consuming data collection and analysis. Labour intensive. Relative subjectivity makes it difficult to generalize results. Analysis may be value-laden.

physiotherapy assistants she chose non-participant overt observation because she felt that participant observation would have been problematic. Because Smith was a physiotherapist herself she was concerned that the assistants would view her as a supervisor rather than a researcher and therefore expect her to act rather than watch. Smith felt this might lead to a loss of trust and equality.

As well as differing in the degree to which the observer participates in the group, observations can differ in the amount of control an observer tries to place on a situation. Exerting control in observation usually involves manufacturing an event or situation in order to see how people react. Millgram's (1963) obedience studies are a classic example of this. Through the use of actors and deception, people were 'pressured' into delivering what they thought were electric shocks to another person. Observations of their reactions were used to argue that people could be manipulated into being 'obedient'. In participant observation the observer does not usually attempt to control what they observe because they are interested in natural situations. In projects where the researcher is a 'complete observer' or non-participant he/she may or may not attempt to control the situation under observation.

With participant observation, the observers are members of the groups they are investigating. This can mean that the observer is observing a group that they naturally belong to or it may mean that they have joined a group that they would not otherwise belong to. The extent of their participation will vary. If you are observing a group that you would naturally belong to then it is likely that your participation is complete. Participant observation is linked very strongly to the qualitative methodology of ethnography (see Chapter 3). With this observation method the observer is interpreting their experience of participation. This requires such personal skills as sensitivity and insight.

Those being observed may or may not know that they are being observed. This knowledge will depend on whether the observer feels it appropriate to be 'honest'. The main advantages of honesty in observational research are that researchers are then able to ask questions in order to clarify observations and have a greater certainty that the people being observed will not object to information being recorded and reported. The main disadvantage of honesty is that if people know they are being observed they are likely to alter their behaviour either consciously or unconsciously and therefore not exhibit 'normal behaviour'. A researcher may be able to be honest and observe natural behaviour by spending considerable time with a group. This way, the researcher becomes 'part of the furniture' and the people may be less affected by his or her presence. There are occasions, however, when people would prefer to be observed by an outsider than by an insider. There can be less personal consequences for someone if they are aware that a stranger is observing them. The outsider will leave the community or group at some point while the insider is more likely to remain a part of that group, carrying information about participants which they may prefer was forgotten.

Whilst observation may aid accuracy and reliability, participation can aid meaning and interpretation. Participation and observation may therefore be seen as conflicting (Peberdy, 1993). This conflict is highlighted when we consider the advantages and disadvantages of participant observation. When researchers consider the advantages of participant observation the focus is usually on the potential to observe people in their natural environment and for the data to be richer in terms of getting at meaning. There are, however, considerable disadvantages. These include the danger of losing objectivity, the observer can be very isolated, the researcher may influence the group's behaviour and complete participants can only study the part of the community to which they belong. It may also be difficult to understand and draw valid inferences from groups that are very different to that which the observer belongs. Finally, participation can be risky if the group activities are criminal or dangerous.

Recording observational data

Whether you are conducting structured or unstructured observations, participating or not participating, it is impossible to record everything (Bell, 1987). This means that observers need to be clear whether they are interested in content, processes, interactions, contributions or some other aspect of behaviour. Observation data can be recorded using check-lists, category systems, field notes, video recording or computer recording.

Check-lists and category systems

Check-lists include a long series of items that can be ticked as present or not present. Compared with check-lists, category systems use a relatively small number of items and attempt to maintain a more or less continuous record. Behaviours that can be coded in a category system include non-verbal behaviours, spatial behaviours (moving towards or away), extra-linguistic behaviours (pace and loudness, interruptions) and linguistic behaviours (content and structure of language).

Category systems are commonly used in structured observations. Observation schedules are employed where each category of behaviour to be observed is defined very carefully. Observation schedules force researchers to be explicit about the concepts they wish to study. A good observation schedule will not allow you to place an observation in more than one category but will allow you to record everything that is considered relevant.

THERAPY EXAMPLE

Galuschka (1987) conducted a structured observational study attempting to evaluate the learning outcomes of two computerized teaching programmes designed to be used with adults who had a severe learning disability. In this study three behavioural categories were identified as being important for providing evidence of learning. These behaviours are identified and defined as follows.

Correct response: The response required from each task. Example: pressing switch or moving joystick.

On-task behaviour: The user pays full attention to the task in hand, attending to their actions and the consequences of those actions. Example: attending to the switch being pressed and watching the consequence of the switch changing on the screen.

Inappropriate behaviour: Any behaviour that is not appropriate to the task in hand. Examples: shrieking, self-injurious behaviour, throwing objects around, attempting to get up and/or leave the room, scratching or biting staff, trying to hide objects and trying to push test objects away.

Coding behaviours like this can allow you to look at interactions such as what happened, who contributed, for how long, what was the nature of the contribution and who talked with whom. When trying to identify pertinent categories of behaviour you can collect information from experts through the use of focus groups or critical incidents or look at other published research sources (Barlow, 1994).

You may be able to use existing coding schemes. The advantage of using someone else's observation schedule is that it is likely to have been tested for reliability and validity. Unfortunately there is a limited number of standardized observation schedules. The number is slowly increasing, however. If you plan to devise your own observation schedule Robson (1993) gives some valuable advice: avoid context-dependent categories where the category depends on the context in which it occurs; explicitly define your categories and make them easy to record; and be exhaustive, covering all possibilities and make your categories mutually exclusive.

No matter how structured or comprehensive our observation schedules are it can be difficult to avoid placing our own interpretation on what we are observing. This biasing effect can be minimized by training a number of observers to use the observation schedule. During the training period disagreements and differences in interpretation can be discussed and the schedule adjusted and refined until the level of agreement between the observers is acceptable. While this type of training can improve reliability, it runs the risk of losing the insights of particularly sensitive researchers. This loss may reduce the validity of the study.

EXERCISE

> A therapist wants to study the behaviour of elderly patients whilst in the day rooms of the hospital. She wants to look at 'engagement' and has devised the following categories: with staff, with other patients, with visitors, alone. What do you think these categories mean? Try to come up with a definition for each one. Now compare your definitions with those of a colleague or friend; how similar or different are your definitions? What are your conclusions from this exercise?

Field notes

Hand-written field notes are frequently employed in semi-structured or unstructured observation. Such notes are often compiled after the observation session has been completed. These notes may include descriptions of events, tentative explanations and interpretation, what the observer has done or said, plus the researcher's own feelings and perceptions.

> **Example of field notes:** An observation of how computers are used with adults who have learning disabilities
> DAY TWO: 27/4/88 Wednesday afternoon
> *Overheard:* The department is going to convert an alcove in one room into a computer room so that it is away from other activities and the clients are not distracted. (Where will the money come from?) The manager and one member of staff got the computer scientist to write software again this week. (Like last week the staff and manager are interacting with the expert.) What kind of software do they want? Adapting old software – want more stimuli, want to know whether the client is paying attention to the screen.
>
> *Observation:* The computer scientist was running the computer sessions with clients, but not in isolation from the staff. The staff were overlooking what was going on in order to see how the clients were progressing. The computer scientist reported back to the staff on progress and the staff filled in the progress sheets. The session was set up especially to make use of the expert's time.

Ideally, observations should be recorded immediately in order to reduce errors and prevent memories becoming blurred. Once the field notes have been completed the observer will often read through them in order to devise categories into which the observations can be placed. This kind of content analysis may run into problems for two reasons. Firstly, if too few categories are devised then the data may be limited, reducing validity. Secondly, if too many categories are devised accuracy may be limited thus reducing reliability.

Video recording

Video recording is possible in a well-financed research project. In order to get optimal data from video recording a number of factors need to be considered. Firstly, the lighting and positioning of equipment need to be checked in order to ensure you have got a clear picture and sound. The recording equipment should be checked to ensure you could record in small units such as microseconds if you needed to. If you need to follow the action then your video camera will need to movable. If you want to follow a sequence of events or sample of variety of situations you may need more than one video camera. If you need to illicit causes and consequences of behaviours then check that your recording equipment will allow the beginnings and endings of events to be easily identified. Finally, you will need to consider whether you hide the cameras or make them very overt. Sometimes it is possible to get the people you are observing to do the filming for you.

THERAPY EXAMPLE

Stillman and McMeeken (1996) describe how they used a video time display to measure gait. They videotaped patients walking and then super-imposed a video time display on to the videotapes. This allowed them to use pause-motion relay in order to obtain measures of walking speed, cadence and stride length. This technique was used to analyse gait under different conditions such as with footwear or bare feet, and with different subject groups, healthy or with head injury, Parkinson's disease, and cerebral palsy. Stillman and McMeeken used the results to assess whether the VTD-based gait analysis can be successfully applied in different situations.

Bottorff (1994) considers the advantages and disadvantages of using videotaped recordings in qualitative research. The main advantage is the permanence of the data that you collect. With the data on videotape you can review events as often as you need, in a variety of ways (real time, slow motion) and compare instances of similar events at different points in time. The main disadvantage is the absence of contextual data beyond that which you have recorded.

Computer recording

Lap-top computers can be very effective in producing observational records while you are in the field or once your data have been recorded using video. For example, Galuschka (1987) used a lap-top computer and a behavioural analysis program to analyse the behaviours of adults with learning disabilities whilst they were using a computer program. The lap-top keys were used to encode behaviours (see Table 6.2). The observer would watch the videos and, when they saw a certain behaviour, pressed the appropriate key on the lap-top. At the end of the observation session the lap-top could produce a printout that gave an analysis of sequences and duration of behaviours.

Table 6.2   Definitions and coding of key behaviours

Person	Behaviour	Lap-top key
Participant	*Correct response:* The response required from each task. Example: pressing switch or moving joystick.	I
	On-task behaviour: The user pays full attention to the task in hand, attending to their actions and the consequences of those actions. Example: attending to the switch being pressed and watching the consequence of the switch changing on the screen.	O
	Inappropriate behaviour: Any behaviour that is not appropriate to the task in hand. Examples: shrieking, self-injurious behaviour, throwing objects around, attempting to get up and/or leave the room, scratching or biting staff, trying to hide objects and trying to push test objects away.	P
Facilitator	*Prompting:* Verbal prompting where the facilitator verbally encourages the user to engage in the task. Example: 'press the switch'. Gestural prompting where the facilitator uses their hands to direct attention or mimic a response. Example: making a swirling action with hand to mimic crayoning on paper.	1
	Reinforcement: Facilitator rewards the user for paying attention or getting a correct response. Examples: verbal congratulations such as 'well done' and 'good boy'; physical congratulations such as patting on the back, cuddling or clapping; production of a tangible reward such as a drink.	Z
	Modelling: Facilitator shows the user what to do by doing the task themselves. Example: showing how to use the joystick by moving it around.	M

You will note that I, O and P are next to one another on the second row of the QWERTY keyboard and can be pressed using the right hand. 1 and z are on the left of the keyboard, 1 at the top and Z at the bottom. These keys can be pressed using the left hand. On the lap-top, the key for 'M' was in the middle of the middle row and can be pressed using either hand. This choice of keys was thought to make encoding the behaviours easy.

Sampling issues in observation studies

The purpose of sampling in observation studies is to ensure that a representative sample of behaviours is obtained, that generalizations can be made from the observed sample to a wider sample and that a detailed understanding of the observed events is gained. The sampling method chosen will depend on the particular research questions posed, as well as the various practical considerations such as time constraints and available resources.

Table 6.3 Dates and times when observations occurred in rooms 1 and 2

Room 1		Room 2	
Date	Time	Date	Time
18.2.86	2.10–3.00	19.2.86	2.25–3.15
20.2.86	2.25–3.15	21.2.86	2.20–3.10
24.2.86	2.35–3.25	25.2.86	2.10–3.00
26.2.86	2.30–3.20	27.2.86	2.20–3.10
28.2.86	2.20–3.10	3.3.86	2.30–3.20

Time sampling

If researchers wish to obtain representative samples of behaviours, it is better for them to observe for short periods on many occasions, than to observe for long periods on a few occasions. If they wish to generalize their data beyond the particular situation they are observing, then the settings must be randomly selected. A systematic time-sampling technique allocates time intervals when behaviour is coded and time intervals when it is not, and these intervals can be randomly assigned.

> **Example of time sampling:** A study of engagement involving elderly patients was conducted in response to staff belief that people were just sitting around all day with nothing to occupy them. The purpose of this study was to look in a structured manner at what patients (mixture of rehabilitation and long-stay clients) did in the day rooms. Two rooms were observed over a period of five days. One fifty-minute observation session was conducted on each of the five days. These sessions occurred at different times in order to provide a representative sample (see Table 6.3).

Time sampling does not allow infrequent events to be recorded. This may be a disadvantage if those infrequent events are important to the research question or topic. The data obtained from time sampling can lack continuity. It can be difficult to ascertain how events are related, particularly if there have been long time intervals between observations. The context in which the behaviour takes place may also be partially lost with time sampling.

Event sampling

With event sampling specific events are recorded as they occur. This sampling method allows more opportunity for unusual or infrequent incidents to be recorded. Event sampling also enables the observer opportunities to record the beginning and end of episodes or events.

> **Example of event sampling:** Figure 6.1 gives an example of the data recorded by Galuschka (1987) using a lap-top computer. As soon as the recording starts, every behaviour is logged. Three types of behaviour (1 = prompting, 0 = on-task, I = correct response) were logged on 23 occasions.

BEH	START	FINISH	DURATN
Day: 1	Client ID: MO		
Observer: JK	Ending time: 166		
Location: Hby	Session No: BL1.1S		
Member of staff: DN			
1	6	7	1
1	8	12	4
1	16	19	3
1	27	27	0
O	28	60	32
O	61	61	0
O	61	62	1
O	62	62	0
O	63	63	0
O	63	64	1
P	64	88	24
O	89	99	10
I	89	94	5
I	96	99	3
O	100	101	1
P	104	116	12
1	118	120	2
I	126	133	7
1	130	134	4
O	134	156	22
I	135	153	18
O	158	166	8
I	159	165	6

Figure 6.1   Computer recording of the event and duration of three observed behaviours.

Pilot studies

Pilot studies allow observers the chance to practice their skills and identify and solve any practical problems. Pilot studies are particularly useful if you are using observational schedules where you have to identify and record predefined categories of behaviour. A pilot study will enable an observer to identify any slightly ambiguous categories or behaviours that have not been defined and categorized but which have been observed as occurring on a frequent or regular basis.

With an observational pilot study you should try to observe people who are as similar to the 'real' research participants as possible. It may also help to discuss your methodology and categories with researchers who have had prior experience of either your observational research technique or your research topic. Conducting pilot studies can help you identify categories, events or behaviours that can be studied further. In addition they help you establish observer consistency (the extent to which an observer obtains the same results measuring the same behaviour on different occasions) and interobserver agreement (the extent to which two or more observers obtain the same results when measuring the same behaviour).

Advantages and disadvantages of observational studies

Observational studies are useful for studying behaviour directly rather than relying on what people say they do. Another advantage is that you can observe people in their natural environment, which provides a context in which to interpret behaviour. Observational studies also require little or no effort on the part of the people who are being observed and can be useful for studying people who are unwilling or unable to participate in other methods such as questionnaires.

The major disadvantages of observational studies are observer effects, observer bias, observer inconsistency and observer drift. Observer effects occur when the mere presence of the observer influences the behaviour of the observed. This is sometimes called the Hawthorne effect. Observer effects can be counteracted by minimal interaction with the group (avoiding eye contact, planning spatial location) or habituation of the group to the observer's presence (repeating your presence to such an extent that it is unrewarding, unnoticed).

Observer bias may occur if the observer misses important phenomenon when recording or allows the coding of the data to be influenced by certain expectations or assumptions. Observer bias might be avoided by videoing the events of interest and asking a third party (someone who does not know your research question) to code the data. This is called 'blind coding'. Endacott (1994) points out that it is possible to use other methods such as interviews to correct unwarranted observer inferences.

Observer consistency is the extent to which an observer obtains the same results when measuring the same behaviour on different occasions. Interobserver agreement is the extent to which two or more observers obtain the same results when measuring the same behaviour. Observer consistency can be achieved through practice and training, perhaps through the use of pilot studies.

However, while an observer may be consistent they may be idiosyncratic in the way they interpret the behavioural codes and categories. Interobserver agreement can be achieved by getting several observers to observe the same behaviours. Consistency and agreement can be measured by looking at the degree to which two sets of measurements are similar. Cohen's Kappa coefficient is frequently used to measure the degree of agreement or concordance.

THERAPY EXAMPLE

Pellecchia (1996) describes a study that attempted to determine the reliability of therapist's assessments of lumbopelvic stabilization (LPS) and base of support (BOS) during manual lifting. Three physiotherapists viewed videotaped observations of 32 subjects lifting a milk crate from floor to waist height and rated both LPS and BOS. She compared the measurements for three pairs (observer 1 with 2, 1 with 3 and observer 2 with 3) using weighted kappa coefficients. The closer the kappa coefficient is to 1, the closer the agreement. Pellecchia used the results to argue for increased reliability in the assessment of patient performance. The results are summarized in Table 6.4.

Table 6.4 Kappa coefficients for three observer pairs who were assessing lumbopelvic stabilization (LPS) and base of support (BOS)

Observer pairs	LPS	BOS
1–2	0.47	0.47
1–3	0.57	0.59
2–3	0.60	0.77

Endacott (1994) argues that it is not always possible or desirable to use two observers in the real situation due to insufficient space to accommodate two observers, increased intrusion, increased observer effect and increased subject anxiety.

Robson (1993) identified a problem he calls 'observer drift'. Observer drift occurs when there are subtle changes in the way an observer uses an observation schedule, due to familiarity or changes in interpretation. Inter-rater reliability and intra-rater checks such as periodic retraining and refreshing can check this.

Key points

1. Observation can be structured or unstructured, participant or non-participant.
2. Check-lists and categories, field notes, video recording and computer recording can be used to record observational data.
3. Sampling enables a representative sample of behaviour to be obtained, from which generalizations can be made.
4. Two types of sampling are time sampling and event sampling.
5. There are advantages and disadvantages of observational studies.
6. Solutions to some of the disadvantages include checking inter-rater and intra-rater reliability.

References

Barlow, S. (1994). Drawing up the schedule for observation. *Nurse Researcher*, **2**, 22–29.

Bell, J. (1987). *Doing Your Research Project*. Open University Press.

Black, N. (1996). Why we need observational studies to evaluate the effectiveness of health care. *British Medical Journal*, **312**, 1215–1218.

Bottorff, J.L. (1994). Using videotaped recordings in qualitative research. In *Critical Issues in Qualitative Research Methods*. (J.M. Morse, ed.), pp. 244–261. Sage Publications.

Endacott, R. (1994). Objectivity in observation. *Nurse Researcher*, **2**, 30–40.

French, S. (1993). *Practical Research: A Guide for Therapists*. Butterworth-Heinemann.

Galuschka, J. (1987). *A behavioural video analysis of computer assisted learning in adults with severe learning difficulties*. Third year project, Psychology Department, Plymouth Polytechnic.

Millgram, S. (1963). A behavioural study of obedience. *Journal of Abnormal and Social Psychology*, **67**, 371–378.

Peberdy, A. (1993). Observing. In *Reflecting on Research Practice: Issues in Health and Social Welfare*. (P. Shakespeare, D. Atkinson and S. French, eds), pp. 47–57. Open University Press.

Pellecchia, G.L. (1996). Visual observation as a method of qualitative analysis of lumbar stabilization and base of support during manual lifting: inter-rater reliability. *Physiotherapy Canada*, **Fall**, 266–270.

Pretzlik, U. (1994). Observational methods and strategies. *Nurse Researcher*, **2**, 13–21.

Robson, C. (1993). *Real World Research: A Resource for Social Scientists and Practitioner-Researchers*. Blackwell.

Smith, S. (1996). Ethnographic inquiry in physiotherapy research. 1. Illuminating the working culture of the physiotherapy assistant. *Physiotherapy*, **82**, 342–348.

Stillman, B. and McMeeken, J. (1996). Use of video time display in determining general gait measures. *Australian Physiotherapy*, **42**, 213–217.

Measuring and measurement tools in research

Measuring and measurement

The research process observes, surveys and measures. This chapter deals with using research to obtain actual measurements. We may want to collect data from simple measurements that reflect activity or the passing of time. For example, we could measure the distance that someone walks in two minutes and then compare that with the distance covered by the same person whilst running. Or we may wish to gather baseline information about someone's physiology, health or well-being so that we can ascertain outcome following a therapy intervention. In order to attain a degree of consistency or reliability over time or across a number of different people it is necessary to standardize the measurement tool and the measurement procedure. Standardized assessment tools are those that have been shown to be valid and reliable in the measurement of specific features of human activity. For example, a tape-measure is a standardized tool in that you can be confident that the distance indicated by one centimetre on your tape-measure will equate to that on all other tape-measures across the world. Not all assessment tools measure numerically. Some assess more abstract elements such as feelings or depression. These tools may not be standardized across the world, as other factors such as culture and race may dictate different standards. Table 7.1 shows how assessment tools have been used to measure different elements of human activity and response.

Levels of measurement

There are four categories of numeric measurement, each giving different levels of information: nominal, ordinal, interval and ratio (Hicks, 1995). Nominal data are characterized by their descriptive nature. This involves a naming category and has no true numeric value. For example, you may categorize participants by sex, either male or female; or you may wish to code responses to a questionnaire – yes or no. You may label categories by letter or number, e.g. group A and group B or group 1 and group 2. Being labelled group 1 does not mean you are inherently better than group 2 in the same way that bus number 17 is no better or worse than bus number 21, it is simply a means of categorization.

Table 7.1 Using different assessment tools to measure different elements of human activity and response

What is being measured	Measurement or assessment tool	Example of use in research
Anatomical structure or movement	Goniometer	Measurement of the effects of massage and infrared radiation on lumbar flexion (Conlon and Maxwell, 1995).
Physiological process	FEV1	Assessment of lung function post lung volume reduction surgery (Grant, 1997).
Disease process–extent	MRI scan	Shoulder anterior instability measured by size of glenoid-laberal tears (Liu *et al.*, 1997).
Disease process–impact	Impact of disease on daily living EORTC QLQ-C30	Impact of cancer on quality of life, body image, future perspective, etc. (Aaronson, 1993).
Pain	Visual analogue scale (VAS) McGill Pain Questionnaire	The clinical role of the VAS for pain (Waterfield and Sim, 1996). Measuring the effect of hydrotherapy for people with low back pain (McIlveen and Robertson, 1998).
Human activity	Test of Visual Perceptual Skills	Measuring the effects of intervention in developmental coordination disorder (Howard, 1997).
	Barthel index	Physiotherapy effects on stroke disability after one year (Warburton, Richardson and Wolfe, 1996).
	Canadian Occupational Performance Measure (COPM)	Evaluation of the impact of primary care occupational therapy (Tyrrell and Burn, 1996).
Psychological morbidity	Hospital Anxiety and Depression Scale (HAD)	Screening for adjustment and depressive disorders in cancer in-patients (Razavi *et al.*, 1990).
Beliefs	Rotter's Internal–External Locus of Control Scale	Investigation of beliefs regarding adjustment to breast cancer (Vinokur *et al.*, 1989).

Ordinal data are more informative as they identify rank rather than category. Imagine a race on the athletics track where competitors cross the line in order – first, second, third and so on. It makes no difference whether athlete two comes in a split second after athlete one and athlete three follows several seconds later. The timings between them are irrelevant to their ranking. Rank order scales are commonly used in research, especially in questionnaires (see Chapter 4).

Interval data give even more information. They are similar to ordinal data in that they identify rank, but the spaces between the ranks are equal. An example of an interval scale is the measurement of temperature in degrees centigrade. The difference in temperature rise between 10 degrees centigrade and 11 degrees centigrade is the same as that between 98 degrees centigrade and 99 degrees centigrade. However, the important point to note is that 0 degrees centigrade does not indicate an absence of temperature, it is simply an easy means of denoting the freezing point of water.

Ratio scales are the most robust numeric data that you can collect. These are similar to interval scales except that they have an absolute zero. Weight is measured using ratio scales. If you weigh out a kilogram of sugar, then remove a kilogram of sugar you will have nothing there!

The level of measurement is important if you intend to subject your data to inferential statistical analysis (see Chapter 9). Inferential statistics divide into two categories: parametric tests and non-parametric tests. Parametric testing is preferable, as it is the more sensitive statistical tool. The conditions for the use of the parametric test include:

1. Data must be interval or ratio.
2. Participants should have been randomly selected.
3. The resultant data should be normally distributed about the mean.

Non-parametric tests may be conducted on interval and ratio data where the other conditions do not apply and also on nominal and ordinal data. Hicks (1995) is a useful reference for researchers wishing to look at statistical analysis in more depth.

Ranking scales

There are three kinds of ranking scales: Likert scales, visual analogue scales and numeric rating scales.

Likert scales

Likert scales are ordinal, ranked scales used frequently in questionnaires as they are quick to complete and easy to analyse. Likert scales comprise a series of 'opinion' statements about an issue (Bowling, 1997). They usually take the form of a five-point scale, and rank someone's opinion from one extreme to the other with a non-committal 'middle ground' statement in the middle. The following choices would be an example:

strongly agree   agree   neither agree nor disagree   disagree   strongly disagree

Some researchers amend the scale to miss out the middle option, as they want to force respondents into having an opinion. This may work very well, but in practice people who really do not feel strongly either way often scribble 'don't know' or 'no preference' on the questionnaire, disrupting analysis.

It is also possible to amend the scale to have seven points, adding the options 'fairly strongly agree' and 'fairly strongly disagree' to the above scale. This is only useful when you expect the majority of respondents to be swayed to one side of the scale and want to ascertain their exact degree of opinion. It is possible to develop your own summated Likert-type rating scale and test it for validity and reliability using the processes set out by Robson (1993). Other forms of amended Likert scaling include visual analogue scales and numeric rating scales.

Visual analogue scales

Visual analogue scales (VASs) are used to measure people's experiences that are individual to them. Often, there is no other quantitative method of ascertaining the impact of that experience. For example, these scales can be used to measure perceived pain, fatigue or effort. These experiences are very personal and a score for one person will not indicate the same level of pain or fatigue for another person. Their use is in the identification of change over time for individuals.

A VAS comprises a carefully drawn 10 cm line (usually horizontal), the ends of which represent the extremes of the experience. For example, on a VAS measuring pain one end may state 'worst pain you can imagine' and at the other end 'pain free'. The participant is asked to indicate their level of pain intensity at the appropriate place on the scale. The researcher then measures from the 'worst' end and notes the numeric score. There is debate as to whether participants should see their previous score before completing a new one. The advantage to seeing the previous score is that the person is then able to judge their perception relative to the first. A VAS may be used in this way to ascertain the effect of a therapy intervention on the person's pain. The VAS will be administered at the start of the treatment session and again at the end. However, there is a case for not showing the previous VAS score between treatments on the premise that the person will not necessarily use comparable starting points.

Because the score depends on accurate measurement of the mark from the end of the scale it is important to ensure that the VAS is exactly 10 centimetres. If you are photocopying VASs ensure that they are not magnified or reduced during the process.

Numeric rating scales

Numeric rating scales are variations of VASs which use numbers as well as adjectives. The scale is marked at equal intervals from 0–10, 0–100, etc. as appropriate. There is no real advantage over the standard VAS although they may reduce measuring and are preferred by some researchers.

Standardized assessments

These are published tests, often well validated and respected, that have become the standard by which more abstract elements such as intelligence or personality are ascertained. These are commonly used in psychology research and it is possible to purchase collections of such tests from The Psychology Corporation and other specialist companies.

Health measurement scales

Health measurement scales are of great value to therapists undertaking research. They fall into four main categories:

1. Functional ability.
2. Mental state.
3. Quality of life, including social health.
4. Disease-specific.

Many books are available to assist the therapy researcher in finding the test most suited to his/her project (Bowling, 1991, 1995; Wade, 1992; Pynsent, 1993; Cole *et al.*, 1995; McDowell and Newell, 1996). These books list the tests, describe their use and identify their validity and reliability.

When choosing a health measurement scale ensure that you are using the right one for the right question and the right participating population. Drummond (1996) suggests the following check-list headings to ensure correct choice:

1. Be clear about what you want to measure. You may want to measure activities of daily living and feel that the Rivermead ADL Assessment fits your requirements, especially as it was first designed to be used both clinically and as a research tool (Cole *et al.*, 1995). However, on closer inspection you may feel that the scaling is too broad and, although this aids reliability, it may not be sensitive enough to ascertain change over your short data collection period.
2. Check whether you are using a valid scale. For example, the Barthel Index is not valid for all populations, e.g. in children.
3. Check whether the scale has been checked for reliability. Can the same results be consistently achieved between test applications and between assessors?
4. Check whether the scale is appropriate to use on your participants. For example, is it appropriate to use self-administered multiple choice questionnaires with people who have a learning disability?
5. Check how much training it takes to become familiar with the scale. Some require special training, e.g. the Gross Motor Performance Measure (Cole *et al.*, 1995).
6. Discuss your choice of scale with a researcher who is familiar with its application and analysis.
7. Consider if another scale would be more appropriate.

Other points to take into consideration include:

1. The cost of the scale: many are copyrighted and some must be purchased or used under licence. Just because a scale is published in a journal this does not give you the automatic right to use it freely. Look for any copyright or trade mark symbol and investigate further before use. Unless a scale is very widely used it is courteous to contact the authors for permission to use it. Most are more than happy to oblige, requiring only acknowledgement in any publications and, perhaps, a copy of your final report.

2. Do not forget that training and explanatory handbooks may also have a cost implication.
3. Making changes to validated scales reduces their validity.
4. Just one test may not be enough to obtain all the information you require. Pilot any tests or scales you intend to use to find out how long they will take to administer and then decide whether your subjects will have the patience and stamina to get through the whole battery. This will also have an impact on researcher time, perhaps limiting the number of subjects that can be entered into the project and increasing data preparation and analysis time.

Therapy outcome measures

Robust therapy outcome measures are used in three main ways: providing evidence of service effectiveness for health commissioners; checking personal clinical effectiveness; and as sensitive research tools to ascertain the impact of therapy intervention on patients and clients (Barnard and Hartigan, 1998). Therapy outcome measures include:

1. Objective measures, e.g. range of movement, distance walked.
2. Subjective measures, e.g. patient: 'I feel better today' or therapist: 'He's walking better today'.
3. Ranked scales, e.g. VAS.
4. Ordinal functional evaluation scales, e.g. TELER™.
5. Health measurement scales, e.g. Functional Independence Measure (FIM).
6. Goal attainment, i.e. using achievement of joint set goals as an outcome measure.
7. Evidence of increased knowledge and adherence to therapy programmes, e.g. diary evidence of stress management.
8. Evidence of change of lifestyle or implementation of coping strategies, e.g. use of taught moving and handling techniques by carers.

To ensure you choose the right outcome measure in your research check that it fulfils the following criteria. It must be:

1. Appropriate, i.e. acceptable, 'do-able'.
2. Valid, i.e. the right outcome for the right job, applied at the right time to the right population.
3. Reliable, i.e. consistency of results.
4. Responsive, i.e. sensitive to any small changes you wish to measure.

Examples from therapy literature

In investigating the long- and short-term effects of Snoezelen® on older people with dementia Baker *et al.* (1997) used several measurement tools to identify changes in behaviour, mood and cognition (see Table 7.2). They were careful to use only those scales appropriate to their population and trained staff in their use. Although the measurement tools used were found to be sensitive to changes in mood and behaviour, the researchers felt that 'some of the very individual benefits . . . were not identified by this study'. It would

Table 7.2 Measurement tools used by Baker *et al.* (1997) to identify changes in mood, behaviour and cognition

Measurement tool	Reference	Used to record or measure
Rehab.	Baker and Hall (1983)	Behaviour in hospital setting
Behaviour and Mood Disturbance Scale	Greene *et al.* (1982)	Behaviour and mood at home (informal scale completed by carers)
Behaviour Rating Scale	Pattie and Gilleard (1979)	Behaviour over time at home (formal scale)
Mini-Mental State Examination	Folstein *et al.* (1975)	Cognition
Cognitive Assessment Scale	Pattie and Gilleard (1979)	Cognition
Interact	Baker and Dowling (1995)	Behaviour during Snoezelen™ sessions

Table 7.3 Measurements used by McIlveen and Robertson (1998) to ascertain the effects of hydrotherapy

Measurement tool	Reference	Used to record or measure
Modified Schöber method	Macrae and Wright (1969)	Lumbar flexion and extension
Hydrogoniometer	Hsieh *et al.* (1983)	Passive straight leg raise
Ranked grading (absent, reduced, normal, increased)	None, common practice	Tendon reflexes
Oxford Rating Scale	Hollis (1976)	Muscle strength
Ranked grading (absent, diminished, normal, increased)	None, common practice	Light touch sensation
Oswestry Low Back Pain Disability Questionnaire	Fairbank *et al.* (1980)	Functional impairment associated with low back pain
McGill Pain Questionnaire	Melzak (1975)	Pain

appear from the discussion of the results that some formal observation of behaviour would have complemented the measurement scale data.

McIlveen and Robertson (1998) used a variety of measurements to ascertain the effects of hydrotherapy in a study of patients presenting with low back or back and leg pain (see Table 7.3). The authors state that they 'chose measures from those that are used conventionally in physiotherapy practice' and note the paucity of published evidence regarding intra- and inter-rater reliability of lower limb neurological tests for this subject group. They describe the reliability trials they undertook to establish the veracity of using these tests in these circumstances. The results of this study show that, although the subjects who had received hydrotherapy showed significant improvement in function over the control group, there was no significant difference between the groups in the other measurements. The authors suggest two possible interpretations of this. Firstly 'that a real difference in [the] other outcome measures might have existed but the sample size was too small for them to reach significance', and secondly 'that hydrotherapy makes little difference to most subjects with low back and leg pain of longer than three months' duration'.

Key points

1. Measurement is vital in research as it allows for comparison between and across different participants and researchers. Different measurement tools are used to assess a variety of human activities ranging from anatomical structure to personal belief.
2. Measurement data can be put into one of four categories: nominal, ordinal, interval or ratio. The more robust the data the more rigorous the statistical test that can be applied to it.
3. Ranking scales are commonly used in research. These include Likert scales, visual analogue scales and numeric rating scales.
4. Health measurement scales are available for assessing the impact of disease, quality of life and beliefs. Many are available and have been tested to ascertain their reliability and validity. It is important to consider both application and participant group when choosing a pre-existing scale.
5. Therapy outcome measures include objective measurement and assessment of function. Increasingly validated health measurement scales such as FIM are being employed.

References

Aaronson, N.K. (1993). The EORTC QLQ-C30: A quality of life instrument for use in international clinical trials in oncology (abstract). *Quality of Life Research*, **2**, 51.

Baker, R. and Dowling, Z. (1995). *Interact. A new measure of response to multisensory environments*. Research publication. Bournemouth Research and Development Support Unit, Institute of Health and Community Studies, Bournemouth University.

Baker, R., Dowling, Z., Wareing, L.A., Dawson, J. and Assey, J. (1997). Snoezelen: its long term and short term effects on older people with dementia. *British Journal of Occupational Therapy*, **60**, 213–218.

Baker, R. and Hall, J. (1983). *Rehab. Rehabilitation Evaluation.* Vine Publishing.

Barnard, S. and Hartigan, G. (in press). *Clinical Audit in Physiotherapy: From Theory Into Practice.* Butterworth-Heinemann.

Bowling, A. (1991). *Measuring Health: A Review of Quality of Life Measurement Scales.* Open University Press.

Bowling, A. (1995). *Measuring Disease.* Open University Press.

Cole, B., Finch, E., Gowland, C., Mayo, N. and Basmajian, J. (1995). *Physical Rehabilitation Outcome Measures.* Canadian Physiotherapy Association.

Conlon, J. and Maxwell, M. (1995). A study of massage and infrared radiation effects on lumbar flexion. *British Journal of Therapy and Rehabilitation,* **2**, 235–238.

Drummond, A. (1996). *Research Methods for Therapists.* Chapman & Hall.

Fairbank, J.C.T., Couper, J., Davies, J.B. and O'Brien, J.P. (1980). The Oswestry Low Back Pain Disability Questionnaire. *Physiotherapy,* **66**, 271–273.

Folstein, M.F., Folstein, S.E. and McHugh, P.R. (1975). 'Mini-Mental State': a practical method for grading the cognitive state of patients for the clinician. *Journal of Psychiatric Research,* **12**, 189–198.

Grant, A. (1997). Lung volume reduction surgery: clarification of the controversy. *Physiotherapy,* **83**, 491–494.

Greene, J.G., Smith, R., Gardiner, M. and Timbury, G.C. (1982). Measuring behavioural disturbance of elderly demented patients in the community and its effect on relatives: a factor analytic study. *Age and Ageing,* **11**, 121–126.

Hicks, C.M. (1995). *Research for Physiotherapists: Project Design and Analysis.* Churchill Livingstone.

Hollis, M. (1976). *Practical Exercise Therapy.* Blackwell Scientific Publications.

Howard, L. (1997). Developmental coordination disorder: can we measure our intervention? *British Journal of Occupational Therapy,* **60**, 219–220.

Hsieh, C.Y., Walker, J.M. and Gillis, K. (1983). Straight leg raising test: comparison of three instruments. *Physical Therapy,* **63**, 1429–1433.

Liu, S.H., Henry, M.H., Nuccion, S., Shapiro, M.S. and Dorey, F. (1996). Diagnosis of glenoid-laberal tears. A comparison between magnetic resonance imaging and clinical examinations. *American Journal of Sports Medicine,* **24**, 149–154.

Macrae, I.F. and Wright, V. (1969). Measurement of back movements. *Annals of Rheumatic Diseases,* **28**, 584–589.

McDowell, I. and Newell, C. (1996). *Measuring Health: A Guide to Rating Scales and Questionnaires.* Oxford University Press.

McIlveen, B. and Robertson, V.J. (1998). A randomised controlled study of the outcome of hydrotherapy for subjects with low back or back and leg pain. *Physiotherapy,* **84**, 17–26.

Melzak, R. (1975). The McGill Pain Questionnaire: major properties and scoring methods. *Pain,* **1**, 277–299.

Pattie, A.H. and Gilleard, C.J. (1979). *Clifton Assessment Procedures for the Elderly.* Hodder and Stoughton.

Pynsent, P., Fairbank, J. and Carr, A. (1993). *Outcome Measures in Orthopaedics.* Butterworth-Heinemann.

Razavi, D., Delvaux, N., Farvacques, C. and Robaye, E. (1990). Screening for adjustment disorders and major depressive disorders in cancer in-patients. *British Journal of Psychiatry,* **156**, 79–83.

Robson, C. (1993). *Real World Research: A Resource for Social Scientists and Practitioner-Researchers.* Blackwell.

Tyrrell, J. and Burn, A. (1996). Evaluating primary care occupational therapy: results from a London primary health-care centre. *British Journal of Therapy and Rehabilitation,* **3**, 380–385.

Vinokur, A.D., Threat, B.A., Caplan, R.D. and Zimmerman, B.L. (1989). Physical and psychological functioning and adjustment to breast cancer. *Cancer,* **63**, 394–405.

Wade, D. (1992). *Measurement in Neurological Rehabilitation*. Oxford University Press.

Warburton, F.G., Richardson, E. and Wolfe, C.D.A. (1996). Physiotherapy effects on disability levels of stroke patients at one year. *British Journal of Therapy and Rehabilitation*, **3**, 673–676.

Waterfield, J. and Sim, J. (1996). Clinical assessment of pain by the visual analogue scale. *British Journal of Therapy and Rehabilitation*, **3**, 94–97.

Complementary reading

Le Roux, A.A. (1993). TELER™: the concept. *Physiotherapy*, **79**, 755–758.

Le Roux, A.A. (1997). *TELER Information Pack*, 4th edn. TELER.

8   Reliability and validity

Truth in research

The need to base clinical intervention on robust research findings is one of the underpinning principles of evidence-based practice. As the movement to ensure that all practice is based on firm evidence gains momentum, it is necessary to look at the very tenet of this assumption. Are the processes of research rigorous and correctly applied? Are the findings of research true? Are the results of research meaningful or generalizable to the patients you treat? Can you take the text of a published article at face value? Truth and reality are perceptions that may vary according to the stance of the researcher and his/her audience. One certainty is knowledge upon which people can form their own opinions. Bork (1992) states that we acquire knowledge in two ways: by faith and by inquiry. Therapists may also argue that they obtain knowledge by experience. Faith is the province of religion and philosophy and therapy experience is gained only through personal engagement with therapeutic practice. Truth as an element of both faith and experience has to be a personal perception. Inquiry, however, needs to be able to stand up to the scrutiny of the inquirer and the wider audience of academics, practitioners and public, it being the acquisition of facts prior to their wider application. The researcher needs to persuade their audiences that the findings of an inquiry are worth paying attention to.

In considering the nature of truth for qualitative research approaches Lincoln (1985) suggests that researchers consider four particular areas.

1. *Truth-value:* The need to establish a degree of confidence about the process and findings of the research.
2. *Applicability:* The need to determine the extent to which research findings about one group of subjects are applicable to any other or whether the findings would have the same applicability in another context.
3. *Consistency:* The extent to which the results may be successfully replicated.
4. *Neutrality:* The need for the results to reflect the findings of the research and not any personal biases or interests of the researcher.

The truth-value of a qualitative study can be ascertained using several methods including prolonged contact with the 'site', persistent observation, discussion with peers, triangulation and feedback from the members of the 'site' being studied. The consistency of a qualitative study can be checked by getting a second party to 'audit' the research trail and check the routes and steps a researcher has taken to get their results and analysis (see Chapters 9 and 11).

In quantitative research approaches to truth-value and consistency are referred to as validity and reliability. In this chapter we will focus on reliability and validity. This focus will allow links to be made with standardized assessments and health measurement scales (see Chapter 7). Looking at the reliability and validity of the research methodology and tools is vital to ensure both the rigour of the research and the certainty of the results. Similarly there is a need to ensure the reliability and validity of the sample if the results are to be at all meaningful in clinical practice (Newell, 1996).

The need for reliability

How would you define a reliable therapist? Probably as someone who is dependable and consistent in their work. We would expect them to turn up at the same time each day and work in a consistent manner. You may have expectations of this therapist based on your knowledge of their reliable nature. For example, if you were going to be late in to work, you may phone knowing with certainty that they would be in to receive your call. Thus, once this therapist has proven their reliability you can start making assumptions based on their regular behaviour. It is the same with research methods and tools. First it is necessary to identify how consistent and dependable a method or tool may be; then, once you are happy, you can start to have some confidence in the results that it measures. Suppose your child makes a stool in the craft, design and technology class at school. The first time you sit on it you may do so rather gingerly. Assuming it supports your weight, you may sit on it with greater confidence the next time. After you have sat on it several times without it collapsing you then sit on it without a second thought and with the certain knowledge that it will bear your weight. Then other people try sitting on the stool. The circumstances may be different. The maker's younger sibling may give it a try. You know they are light enough to sit on it without problems, but what happens when they kick against the legs? A heavier person will need to start again with the same careful approach as you did. The same 'try it and see' approaches also have to be gone through when deciding which method and tool to use in a research project. This applies throughout the research process. Papers reporting research should establish the credibility of the process and indicate the level of transferability of the findings, allowing the reader to make a judgement as to whether the technique can be integrated into clinical practice (Gliner, 1994).

Definitions of reliability

Reliability is the extent to which you can rely on the results obtained from an instrument (DePoy and Gitlin, 1993). It refers to the ability to produce consistent results and to maintain consistent results on different occasions where there is no evidence of change (Bowling, 1995). It is necessary to ensure the reliability of the research tools, the information gathering tests and the application of those tools or tests. In ensuring the reliability of the tools you must be able to trust your measuring tool or instrument. A stretchy tape-measure will not give consistent or dependable results when measuring leg length. In ensuring the reliability of tests you must be certain that a test will give consistent results in every area that you wish to use it. In ensuring reliability of application you must adhere to a specific measurement protocol. Measuring ankle swelling at the level of the medial malleolus will give a different result to that gained by measuring the same ankle with the same tape-measure two centimetres above the medial malleolus. Similarly, questionnaires need to be administered in the same way to each respondent if the results are to be consistent.

Testing reliability

Researchers and clinicians are looking for a high degree of reliability in their clinical measurement. There is always the likelihood of some error creeping into the measurement. This can be stated as a formula:

observed score = true score + error

The reliability of a measurement can be expressed as:

$$\text{Reliability} = \frac{\text{variation around a true score}}{\text{variation around an observed score}}$$

The result of this equation calculated mathematically is known as the reliability coefficient. The scores of this coefficient range from 0 to 1. The higher the coefficient, the more reliable is the measurement. The reliability of standardized assessment tools such as health measurement scales can be obtained from the literature (Bowling, 1991, 1995; McDowell and Newell, 1996). The reliability of equipment and other measurement hardware should be available from the manufacturers.

Bowling (1997, p. 130) states that 'Certain parameters . . . need to be assessed before an instrument can be judged to be reliable'. These include test–retest reliability, inter-rater reliability, parallel forms and internal consistency. Test–retest reliability is the extent to which one rater obtains consistency in a repeated measurement. To prevent the tester from remembering the result, a 'blinded' measuring tool may be used or enough time may be allowed to elapse to allow the rater to forget their original measurement.

Inter-rater reliability is the extent to which two different raters obtain the same result from the same test. For example, two independent researchers may administer the Functional Independence Measure to the same client. Similar or identical results indicate a high inter-rater reliability.

Parallel (alternate) forms involves a comparison of two forms of the same test or two tests developed in parallel that measure the same attribute. A high correlation between the scores indicates a reliable test.

Internal consistency involves tests for homogeneity and includes the split-half test in which part of a measurement scale measuring one entity is split, usually into odd numbered and even numbered responses, and compared for consistency of response. A high level of agreement between the two halves of the scale indicates a good degree of internal consistency.

Reliability may be described statistically. The type of statistical test used will depend on the reliability parameter (e.g. test–retest, inter-rater, etc.) and data type (i.e. nominal, ordinal, interval, ratio). Readers are referred to Bowling (1997) and McDowell and Newell (1996) for further information.

Examples from the literature of reliability testing

The following therapy examples show how standardized tests and clinical procedures may be investigated for reliability and illustrate the rigorous methods used to establish this. Statistical analyses of the results give the evidence of their reliability.

Connelly, Stevenson and Vandervoort (1996) assessed between and within-rater reliability of walking tests in an elderly, frail population. The study investigated the inter-rater and intra-rater reliability of the timed 10-metre walk test and the 2-minute walk test in a population of 20 frail, elderly people. Each participant undertook three trials of the timed 10-metre walk test on two consecutive days for two different physiotherapy raters. One week later, the same elderly people undertook one 2-minute walk test for each physiotherapy rater, again on two consecutive days. Care was taken to ensure consistency of application of the tests between and within participants. The Intraclass Correlation Coefficients were calculated, ranging from 0.75 to 0.93 for the timed 10-metre test and 0.82 to 0.95 for the 2-minute walk test. These results indicate that, with this group, therapists can obtain reproducible values for both tests when comparing between more than one clinically experienced rater and on more than one occasion.

McKenzie and Taylor (1997) looked at inter-rater and intra-rater reliability in physiotherapists' ability to locate spinal levels by palpation. Three physiotherapists palpated five normal subjects five times to assess intra-therapist reliability. Different spinal levels were randomly allocated. In order to assess inter-therapist reliability fourteen physiotherapists palpated five normal subjects once each. Inter-rater reliability was considered only fair (kappa = 0.28) but good intra-rater reliability was noted (kappa ranging from 0.61 to 0.90). These results indicate a high level of consistency for therapists palpating the same spinal level within the same session but suggest less reliability between therapists.

The need for validity

Therapists are well aware of the need for validity. Using valid clinical measurement is the basis of effective clinical practice (Gould, 1994). Of course you would not measure an attribute such as weight with a tape-measure but this distinction becomes much less obvious when measuring perceptions or feelings or quality of life. A quality of life scale may be perfectly valid for use in one population, but would it be valid for use in another population from another culture? Would it ask the right questions in the right way with the right degree of sensitivity? French (1993) states that validity is much more difficult to ascertain than reliability as it is concerned with the very nature of reality. Cole *et al.* (1995) state that, when selecting a particular measurement tool, validity is the most important consideration. However, validity can only be assigned to a tool after it has been satisfactorily and repeatedly tested on the population for which it has been designed (Bowling, 1997). Testing for validity involves looking at the predictive quality of the tool and seeking evidence of correlation with other similar tools or scales. For example, in a study by Wylie and White (1964) the Barthel Index was shown to successfully predict mortality and length of hospital stay for people with strokes when compared with the independent predictions of a physician.

Definitions of validity

Validity may be defined as 'the extent to which a test measures what it is intended to measure' (Cole *et al.*, 1995, p. 29). It implies appropriateness, truthfulness, authenticity and effectiveness (Payton, 1988). The results of research need to be validated to show that the results are attributable to the intervention being tested rather than any extraneous event (internal validity) and that the results are generalizable beyond the sample researched (external validity).

Testing validity

Validity comprises many components, the implications of which need to be addressed when deciding how to gather research data. We will briefly outline face validity, content validity, criterion validity and construct validity.

Face validity is the subjective assessment of the measurement tool to ensure that it is relevant and unambiguous. For example, questionnaires should be looked at carefully to ensure that the questions are clear and unambiguous.

Content validity is similar to face validity but this time you are looking at the concepts and thinking behind the tool to ensure that it has the potential to obtain the right information. For example, does your questionnaire have the capacity to answer your research question?

Criterion validity is assessed on the ability of a test to correlate with other similar tools (concurrent validity) and its ability to predict outcome (predictive validity). For example, the Nottingham Health Profile has been found to correlate moderately well with Goldberg's General Health Questionnaire and well with clinical judgements of morbidity and prognosis (Bowling, 1991).

Cole *et al.* (1995, p. 30) state that construct validity is the extent to which 'the scores obtained concur with the underlying theories relating to the content' (see validity examples).

Ensuring the validity of your study

In order to ensure the validity of your study it is important to assess the possible threats to validity. Threats to validity include history, testing, maturation, mortality and setting.

History is a threat to validity because unexpected life changes may be responsible for observed changes. For example, becoming a big lottery winner may influence previously held views about private medical care.

Testing threatens validity because research participants may improve on their testing because of learning effects and not because of any inherent improvement. For example, healthy subjects involved in a study investigating the energy cost of using different walking aids may improve during the test simply because they get used to the equipment. Similarly, they may perceive a higher energy cost towards the end of testing, not because the task is any harder, but because they are becoming fatigued.

Maturation is the effect of developmental changes over time. For example, in a longitudinal study, children's coordination will improve, not necessarily because they are working hard at their exercise programme but because normal neurological development is taking place.

Participants may drop out of a study, skewing the results (mortality). For example, you may be very pleased with the results of a training programme for people with chronic pain. However, you need to be aware that people dropping out of the study may be those who are dissatisfied with the intervention and this has an important bearing on the project results.

It is only possible to generalize results to other similar settings and populations. For example, the levels of satisfaction of parents of disabled children in special schools are not automatically generalizable to the parents of disabled children in mainstream schools.

The validity of health measurement scales has often been formally tested and this information can be found in the literature, specifically in health measurement scale books such as those by Bowling (1991, 1995) and McDowell and Newell (1996). The appropriateness of your methodology and measurement tool can often be decided in discussion with colleagues who have previous clinical or research experience in this area. Remember that different methodologies and tools are appropriate for use in different areas and with different populations.

Examples from the literature of validity testing

Tabatabainia, Ziviani and Maas (1995) tested the construct validity of the Bruininks–Oseretsky Test of Motor Proficiency and the Peabody Developmental Motor Scales. Both tests were administered to 40 children aged between 4.5 and 5.5 years. Factor analysis of the subsets failed to support the original subdivision of both tests into fine and gross motor composites, although it did suggest the existence of one other factor, 'general motor proficiency', underlying the structure of both test subsets. The authors contend that it is therefore misleading to claim subdivision of these tests into gross and fine motor composites.

Harris and Daniels (1996) set out to assess the content validity of the Harris Infant Neuromotor Test, a screening tool to detect early signs of cognitive and neuromotor delay in infants with known risk factors. An international panel of 26 multi-disciplinary experts was convened to review, assess and suggest modifications for the test. A validity questionnaire was developed, designed in three parts relating to the three parts of the test. Individual items within each part were sent to the experts. Data were analysed using descriptive statistics. Overall, the experts agreed that the items on the test were 'clearly worded and free from cultural bias'. Feedback from the experts enabled additional questions to be added and others to be modified. The information from the experts suggested that the content of the Harris Infant Neuromotor Test is 'representative of early neuromotor behaviours that can discriminate infants with neuromotor impairments from those who will develop typically'. Less support was demonstrated for the test's ability to discriminate early cognitive delays.

The relationship between reliability and validity

If you were to weigh yourself on the bathroom scales on a daily basis you would note the normal fluctuations of weight over time. These scales probably give a reliable measurement. After Christmas they register a few more pounds and after the pre-summer holiday diet they register a few less. Bathroom scales are an eminently valid tool for this task. It would certainly not be valid nor appropriate to use the kitchen scales or a tape-measure! However, if you then decide to weigh yourself on another set of scales at the gym you may be surprised to notice a difference in your weight. This is not because you have gained a couple of pounds *en route*; rather your bathroom scales are not 'zeroed' accurately, giving a false reading. Thus, it is entirely possible to have an instrument that is utterly reliable yet not truly valid. Similarly it is quite possible to have an instrument that is totally valid yet unreliable. One does not ensure nor preclude the other. For example, it is entirely valid to ask patients their feelings about the therapy they received in a patient satisfaction survey. However, if the treating therapist were to ask these questions the answers may be unreliable, as the patients could feel inhibited about telling the truth. Researchers aim to ensure both the reliability and validity of their methodology, measuring instruments, application and sample, otherwise the results cannot be said to be robust and are lacking in truthfulness and generalizability.

Key points

1. Unless research is based in truth it cannot be said to be reliable or valid.
2. Reliability is the extent to which you can rely on the results of your methodology and measurement tool.
3. Reliability can be tested in various ways, e.g. for inter-rater reliability, test–retest reliability and internal consistency. Reliability can be calculated statistically. Many standardized tests and health measurement scales have been tested in this way. This information needs to be taken into account when deciding on the most appropriate tool for your study.

4. Validity is the extent to which a test measures what it is designed to measure.

5. Different aspects of validity, e.g. face validity, content validity and criterion validity, can be tested to ascertain the appropriateness, truthfulness and authenticity of the tool.

6. Validity can be threatened by many factors including learning effect, developmental maturation and a failure to take all appropriate factors such as the characteristics of a sample population into account.

7. Ensure the validity of your study through discussion with experts and checking validity studies in the literature.

8. A reliable scale is not always a valid scale. Similarly, a valid scale is not automatically a reliable scale.

References

Bork, C.E. (1992). *Research in Physical Therapy*. Lippincott Company.

Bowling, A. (1991). *Measuring Health: A Review of Quality of Life Measurement Scales*. Open University Press.

Bowling, A. (1995). *Measuring Disease*. Open University Press.

Bowling, A. (1997). *Research Methods in Health: Investigating Health and Health Services*. Open University Press.

Cole, B., Finch, E., Gowland, C., Mayo, N. and Basmajian, J. (1995). *Physical Rehabilitation Outcome Measures*. Canadian Physiotherapy Association.

Connelly, D.M., Stevenson, T.J. and Vandervoort, A.A. (1996). Between and within-rater reliability of walking tests in an elderly frail population. *Physiotherapy Canada*, **48**, 47–51.

DePoy, E. and Gitlin, L.N. (1993). *Introduction to Research: Multiple Strategies for Health and Human Services*. Mosby.

French, S. (1993). *Practical Research: A Guide for Therapists*. Butterworth-Heinemann.

Gliner, J.A. (1994). Reviewing qualitative research: proposed criteria for fairness and rigour. *Occupational Therapy Journal of Research*, **14**, 78–90.

Gould, A. (1994). The issue of measurement validity in health-care research. *British Journal of Therapy and Rehabilitation*, **1**, 99–103.

Harris, S.R. and Daniels, L.E. (1996). Content validity of the Harris Infant Neuromotor Test. *Physical Therapy*, **76**, 727–736.

Lincoln, Y.S. (1985). *Naturalistic Inquiry*. Sage Publications.

McDowell, I. and Newell, C. (1996). *Measuring Health: A Guide to Rating Scales and Questionnaires*. Oxford University Press.

McKenzie, A.M. and Taylor, N.F. (1997). Can physiotherapists locate lumbar spinal levels by palpation? *Physiotherapy*, **83**, 235–239.

Newell, R. (1996). The reliability and validity of samples. *Nurse Researcher*, **3**, 16–26.

Payton, O.D. (1988). *Research: The Validation of Clinical Practice*. F.A. Davis Company.

Tabatabainia, M.M., Ziviani, J. and Maas, F. (1995). Construct validity of the Bruininks–Oseretsky Test of Motor Proficiency and the Peabody Developmental Motor Scales. *Australian Occupational Therapy Journal*, **42**, 3–13.

Wylie, C.M. and White, B.K. (1964). A measure of disability. *Archives of Environmental Health*, **8**, 834–839.

Complementary reading

Sim, J. (1995). The external validity of group comparative and single system studies. *Physiotherapy*, **81**, 263–270.

Sim, J. and Arnell, P. (1993). Measurement validity in physical therapy research. *Physical Therapy*, **73**, 102–110.

Titchen, A. (1995). Issues of validity in action research. *Nurse Researcher*, **2**, 38–59.

9 Principles of analysing data

The purpose of data analysis

In our experience data analysis can be the least planned stage of a research project. We can spend ages agonizing over the design and approach, yet put little thought into how we are going to analyse the data and what we hope to achieve through data analysis. Data analysis involves making sense of the information collected in order to obtain explanations. How we try to do that will depend on whether our data are of a quantitative or qualitative kind.

In qualitative research the explanations might be varied. In considering the outcomes of qualitative research, Mason (1996) distinguished between five different kinds of explanations that qualitative data analysis might produce: comparative, developmental, descriptive, predictive and theoretical. A comparative explanation compares social phenomena, processes, locations and meanings. A developmental explanation traces and accounts for the development of social phenomena, processes and change. This involves a story or narrative. A descriptive explanation constructs an explanatory account of what is going on in a particular situation. A predictive explanation is based on the principle that you may be able to predict what might happen in the future under similar conditions. Finally, a theoretical explanation seeks a wider relevance to other explanatory bodies of knowledge or social interpretation.

There are two major functions of quantitative data analysis. The first function is to describe and summarize what has been found. The second function is to try and explain what caused the results. Explanations are sought by testing predictions about the effect certain interventions will have on the measurements made. Part of this testing involves making inferences about whether the results are due to chance or to a significant effect of the intervention.

Qualitative data analysis

Providing a general outline of how to conduct qualitative data analysis is a nigh on impossible task. This is because each methodology approaches analysis in a slightly different way. The approach may be different in terms of the process or the outcomes. Whilst certain steps or tasks can be identified, these need to be viewed carefully because for some methodologies the steps will be sequential and for others they will be concurrent.

Preparing your data

Before any analysis can take place the data must be prepared. For observations and untaped interviews this may involve typing up field notes, and for taped interviews this will involve listening to and transcribing the tapes. Part of the typing and transcription will involve identifying who did or said what and making identifiable names anonymous. Depending on your mode of analysis, word-processed notes and transcriptions may then be imported into a computer program.

Coding your data

The coding of data involves organizing and retrieving sections of text or elements of data for the purpose of further analysis or manipulation. Coding links different segments or instances in the data. Coding may involve looking at all of your data or just discrete parts of it (Mason, 1996). For example, coding may involve a search for the common, using the same 'lens' to search across all the data (cross-sectional indexing). Alternatively, coding may involve a search for something in particular, in which case you may not necessarily use the same 'lens' across the whole data set (non-cross-sectional indexing).

The purpose of coding is to bring fragments of text together in order to create either themes or categories that we define as having a common property or element. If we view a theme as a general topic or idea, then coding may not incorporate the whole data set in the identification of a theme. If we view a category as a class or division into which things might be sorted or distributed, then the purpose of coding in this instance may be to create categories into which the whole data set may be sorted.

Interpreting your data

If the result of coding is the identification of themes, the researcher may simply describe the emergent themes or go one step further and try to interpret them by reorganizing them. If the result of coding is the identification of categories, the researcher may describe these categories (and subcategories) or go further and try to link them in some way. For example, in grounded theory, coding is seen as a two-step process. The first step is called 'open coding' and is seen as a process of breaking down. Categories are gradually built up through a process of comparing and categorizing. The second step is called 'axial coding' and involves putting the data back together in new ways by making connections between categories.

> **Example of linking categories:** A researcher conducts an interview with a lady called Alice Gibson, who has been working in a housing department for five years. Four months ago she gained promotion, which she is finding difficult and is thinking of giving up work altogether. As the interview progresses Alice reveals that she loves her work but is finding it difficult to balance this with her role as wife and mother. From the interview the researcher identifies a key category that they call Stress. Having identified this category the researcher is able to identify and link other categories such as the conditions that give rise to stress, the context in which it is

embedded, the strategies by which it is handled or managed and the consequences of those strategies (see Figure 9.1).

Checking your interpretation

In qualitative research a lot of emphasis is placed on checking or verifying your analysis of the data. Checking or verifying your analysis can help to counter the criticisms of subjectivity and bias that are often thrown at qualitative researchers. You can check your analysis by asking a colleague or participant to read your data and validate or confirm the themes or categories you have identified. Alternatively, you may ask a third party to read your data, devise their own themes and categories and then compare them with the themes and categories that you have identified. In the event that there are huge discrepancies or disagreements between the researcher and those trying to verify the analysis, then it may be useful to revisit your field notes, coding and transcription notes in order to revisit the reasons for your decisions and judgements (see Chapter 11).

Manual and computer analysis of qualitative data

Analysing qualitative data by hand may involve manual indexing or the construction of diagrams and charts. If you plan to index your data manually then your first task is to decide what counts as data. You then read and scrutinize your data in order to apply indexing or

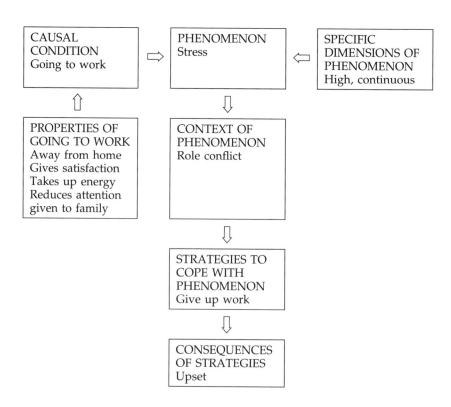

Figure 9.1 Making connections.

category codes to appropriate chunks of text. You might do this in margins alongside the text or by creating subheadings at relevant points in the text. You are advised to keep a separate record of the location of each entry of the code or label (identifiers), e.g. page number, paragraph line number. To retrieve the information you can use the indices to locate whatever it is you want in the data (like the index of a book).

Diagrams and charts can be constructed as a tool in their own right or to aid cross-sectional and non-cross-sectional forms of organization. They identify and represent what you see as the key elements of a particular and holistic part of your data. Diagrams may be easier and quicker to read when dealing with such things as spatial layout or sequences of interaction. You may not show a diagram in your report, but it can influence your thinking and analysis, when spotting connections, for example. Most diagrams are two-dimensional, which may restrict their explanatory potential. Diagrams can be literal (spatial layout), interpretative (cognitive map) or reflexive (your own reasoning process).

Example of the use of diagrams: After extensive observations and interviews Seale (1993) developed an extended metaphor of a cruciform to describe microcomputer use in adult special education. She represented this metaphor by the use of a diagram (see Figure 9.2). Seale explained her diagram by drawing a comparison with creating a cross out of two pieces of wood. One obvious method is to place one piece vertically and the other across it horizontally. One might secure the two pieces together with a nail in the middle. Without the nail the cross would collapse. Applying this idea to microcomputer use in adult special education, Seale argued that the 'nail' that secures effective microcomputer use is planning and decision-making. Without effective planning in a centre, resources, staff involvement, support systems and the microcomputer itself would be neglected.

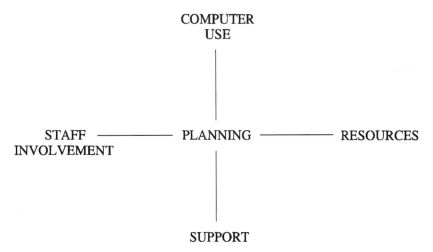

Figure 9.2   The cruciform as a metaphor to describe microcomputer use.

Table 9.1   Distinguishing between different types of computer analysis

Text retrieval	Description/analysis	Theory building
Retrieves words and phrases.	Attaches codes to segments of text.	Develops an indexing system.
Finds individual words or places words into specified categories.	Searches for text segments according to codes and assembles them.	Searches for codes and builds an index system in a separate data base.
Example: GOfer	Example: Ethnograph	Example:Nud.IST

Tesch (1990) outlines how computer programs can help in the analysis of qualitative data. Computer analysis may involve text retrieval, coding segments of text or developing an index system (see Table 9.1). Indexing by computer involves entering the data into the computer in a form that the software package will accept. You then read the texts and use the system provided by the software for entering indexing or category codes. The computer cannot create the codes for you, unless your codes are very literal such as particular words that the computer could search for.

Text retrieval might involve a search program or a content analysis program. Search programs find individual words and phrases in text (across many files). They are extremely fast but require you to index your files first. Content analysis programs take inventories of the words contained in the text. These programs have dictionaries that have rules for assigning words to categories. The program will use these rules to assign the words in the text to different categories. Text retrieval programs may assist analysis by:

1. Making lists of all the different words in one or more document.
2. Counting the frequency of each unique word.
3. Comparing the word lists of different documents.
4. Locating specified words in one or several documents.
5. Constructing indices.
6. Assigning words in the text to categories in one or more document.
7. Extracting specified words from a text together with the words preceding and succeeding each occurrence.
8. Extracting words from a text together with the sentences or paragraphs in which each occurs.
9. Extracting words from a text together with a user-selected context (cut and paste).

Description or analysis programs search sections of text according to predetermined codes. The program will indicate the beginning and end of a text segment, attach the appropriate code-word to the segment and bring together all the segments with the same code by searching and sorting. Such programs allow you to enhance analysis by:

1. Searching for multiple codes.
2. Searching for a particular sequence of codes.
3. Searching selectively.
4. Counting the frequency of the occurrence of codes.

Theory building programs create a separate data base for the categories, which are put in a tree-like structure with information about the associated segments of text. These programs work by searching for co-occurring or overlapping coding within data segments or within entire files and then searching for counter-evidence.

Advantages of using computers to analyse qualitative data include quick and efficient information retrieval and the ability to trace connections, overlaps and relationships. But while computer programs do the cutting, pasting and retrieval of field notes for you, you still need to code the material. Bryman and Burgess (1994) argue that computers simply ease the operations that follow on after coding has been done. Computers cannot substitute for 'the imagination' that is argued to be a necessary ingredient of analysis. There is also concern regarding how far the different programs might condition the analysis that is undertaken. It would probably be wise to speak to other researchers who have used computer analysis to find out the pros and cons of each program.

Quantitative data analysis

There are two major functions of quantitative data analysis. The first function is to describe and summarize, and is achieved through the use of descriptive statistics. The second function is to make inferences and produce explanations, and is achieved through the use of inferential statistics.

Descriptive statistics

Raw data can be unmanageable due to their mass and bulk. It can be difficult to see the important implications of raw data without the use of summarizing tools. Descriptive statistics allow us to summarize the bulk of our raw data. Descriptive statistics summarize data in two ways: they can provide a measure of central tendency or a measure of dispersion. Measures of central tendency give us an indication of what the average or typical score looks like. Measures of dispersion give an indication of how far from the average the scores are spread. There are three measures of central tendency, the mean, the median and the mode.

The mean is known as the arithmetic average. It is calculated by dividing the number of scores by the sum of the data. The mean is the most commonly used average. It is useful if the numbers cluster together. Every score is involved in the calculation of a mean.

Example: Marks on a test (maximum mark is 10)

5   7   4   8   6

Mean $= 30/5 = 6$

A disadvantage of the mean is that if there are extreme scores that are widely spread then the mean can be very misleading. For example scores of 5, 1, 60, 4 and 3 will produce a mean of 14.6, which is unrepresentative of the majority of the scores.

The mode is the score that occurs most frequently. The mode is useful for describing nominal data. The mode may misrepresent the sample as a whole and can be unstable. It can change if just one of the numbers in the set changes, or it may not be altered by radical changes to a lot of scores. There can be several modes in a set of numbers, in which case the modes will need summarizing themselves, and this reduces the use of the mode as a descriptive statistic.

Example:

12   3   3   24   27   2   3   3

Mode = 3

The median is the middle score in a group of scores. The median is less effected by extreme scores than the mean. It is calculated by arranging the scores in numerical order and then finding the score that is in the centre. If there is an even number of scores, the mean of the two central scores becomes the median. Disadvantages of the median include the fact that it can be tedious to order a large list of numbers. The median is also unstable; if one of the central scores moves a little, the median changes. Alternatively, the median may not be altered by radical changes to a lot of scores.

Example:

2   3   5   6   7   9   11   13   17

Median = 7 (four scores below, four scores above)

There are two main measures of dispersion, the range and the standard deviation. The range of a set of scores can be obtained by calculating the difference between the lowest and highest score. The range can give useful information when an average is not indicating a difference between two sets of scores.

Example:

Set 1

21   30   45   50   60   70   85   95

Mean = 57

Range = 95–21 = 74

Set 2

54   55   56   57   57   58   59   60

Mean = 57

Range = 60–54 = 6

Deviation provides information about the extent each score deviates from the mean while variance is the total amount that a set of scores deviates from the mean. Variance is calculated by squaring each deviation score and adding the results up. Standard deviation is the average amount of deviation and is calculated by dividing the variance by the total number of scores and taking the square root of the result:

$$SD = \sqrt{\frac{\sum(x - \bar{x})^2}{N - 1}}$$

where $\bar{x} =$ mean of the group of scores and $N =$ total number of scores.

Example:

21   30   45   50   60   70   85   95

Mean $= 57$
Range $= 74$
SD $= 25.7$

If the standard deviation of a group of scores is large, the scores are widely distributed with many scores occurring a long way from the mean. If the standard deviation of a group of scores is small, the scores are closely clustered and most occur very close to the mean. The lowest standard deviation is 0, indicating no deviation at all; all the scores are identical. The standard deviation is more stable than the range because information from every score is obtained in order to calculate it.

EXERCISE

The data in Table 9.2 have been obtained from 119 therapy students. They were asked to indicate on a scale of 1 to 5 the extent to which they thought therapists and doctors would be involved in a number of research activities (1 being highly probable, 5 being most unlikely).

1. Summarize the main findings from this table – are there any differences between responses for therapists and doctors and, if so, where do they lie?
2. Which do you think is the most informative/meaningful average to use?
3. How does the information from the range and standard deviation supplement that from the averages?
4. Can this information be presented in any format other than a table?
5. What qualitative data do you think it would it be useful to have in order to gain a wider understanding of these results?

Inferential statistics

Descriptive statistics simply summarize what you have found – they make no attempt to go beyond the data obtained and make predictions as to whether the results are likely to be significant. They do not explain what caused the results. Inferential statistics, on the other hand, test

Table 9.2 Descriptive data from statements regarding the probability of therapists and doctors being involved in a number of research activities

	Mean TH	Mean DOC	Med. TH	Med. DOC	Mode TH	Mode DOC	Range TH	Range DOC	Stand. dev. TH	Stand. dev. DOC
Collecting clinical data	2.09	2.23	2	2	1	2	5	5	1.08	1.11
Analysing clinical data	2.27	2.12	2	2	2	2	4	5	1.03	1.00
Applying research findings to practice	1.97	2.03	2	2	2	2	5	5	0.96	1.04
Generating research ideas	2.95	2.52	3	3	3	3	4	5	0.93	1.02
Reading non-research journal articles	2.07	2.21	2	2	1	2	5	5	1.03	1.08
Reading research journal articles	1.70	1.915	2	2	1	1	5	5	0.91	1.08
Attending conferences and workshops	1.70	1.915	2	2	1	2	5	5	0.90	1.02
Speaking at conferences and workshops	2.73	2.1	3	2	3	2	3	5	0.92	1.05
Being a research assistant or collaborator	3.14	3.07	3	3	3	3	5	5	0.95	1.15
Being an independent or principal researcher	3.44	2.73	4	3	4	3	5	5	1.06	1.08
Publishing non-research articles	3.42	2.80	3	3	3	3	5	5	1.05	1.16
Publishing research articles	3.43	2.57	3	3	3	3	5	5	1.07	1.19

Med. = median; Stand. dev. = standard deviation; TH = therapist; DOC = doctor.

predictions (hypotheses) that are made and allow inferences from the data as to whether the data are significant or due to chance factors.

A hypothesis operationalizes what a study is about. It predicts a relationship between two or more variables, states the relationship to be either a difference or an association (correlation) and states the direction of the relationship.

Variables are events that vary in the experimental situation. There are two kinds of variables: independent and dependent. An independent variable is a variable that the researcher manipulates and varies in different conditions. The conditions are set up independently before the study begins (e.g. crutches or no crutches, antidepressant drug A or drug B). A dependent variable is a variable that is dependent on the way in which the experimenter manipulates the independent variable. The results that the researcher collects are measures of the dependent variable (e.g. ability to walk, level of depression).

The independent variable elicits an effect on the dependent variable. There are lots of other things, however, that might affect the results of an experiment apart from the independent variable. Unless these things are controlled for in some way, ensuring that any effect they have is the same in both conditions, we may have no way of knowing whether any difference in the dependent variable was due to the independent variable or to these other factors. We therefore need to design experiments that avoid as many extraneous variables as possible.

In order to assess whether a hypothesis that is looking at differences is true or not a researcher can manipulate an independent variable to see whether it has an effect on the dependent variable. Subjects can be allocated to circumstances that represent the different conditions of the independent variable. The researcher then tests whether there is a difference in the measurements or dependent variables obtained from these different conditions.

> **Example:**
> Hypothesis: Exposure to treatment will improve mobility.
> Independent variable: Treatment scheme to improve mobility.
> Dependent variable: Scores on a mobility assessment.
> Conditions: Treatment/no treatment.

If the mobility assessment scores are significantly higher for those who received treatment than for those who did not, the researcher can claim that his prediction has been proved. That is, there is a difference between the treatment and control condition.

There are times when experimenters are less interested in predicting differences in behaviours as a result of an independent variable; instead they want to investigate whether variables are associated or correlated together. For example, in order to test the hypothesis that mobility and intelligence are associated, all the subjects would be given a mobility test and an intelligence test. But neither of the variables would be the dependent variable or the independent variable. The researcher would take measures of both variables in order to see whether those who score highly on mobility also score highly on intelligence, while those who score less well in mobility also score less well on the intelligence test.

The direction of a relationship can be stated in a hypothesis as either unidirectional or bidirectional. A unidirectional (one-tailed) hypothesis makes a prediction in one particular direction. For example, practice on intelligence tests will increase mobility. A bidirectional (two-tailed) hypothesis makes a prediction that the effect of an independent variable may go in either direction. For example, practice on intelligence tests will result in either improved or worsened mobility.

It is obviously preferable to be able to give an explanation of human behaviour in terms of predicting behaviour in one direction rather than state vaguely that there will be an effect of some kind in either direction. However, there are times, particularly during the more exploratory phase of a research programme, when you might just want to try out whether a variable has any effect. For example, whether improving intelligence has any good or bad effect on mobility levels.

In order to analyse an experiment using inferential statistics it must pose a hypothesis that tests predictions and involves empirical comparisons. For example, the hypothesis 'exercise and diet is the best way to lose weight' is not testable because there is no sense of what exercise and diet are being compared with. A more testable hypothesis might be 'exercise and diet result in more weight loss than diet alone'.

A hypothesis must also state exactly what variables make up the relationship or difference. For example, the hypothesis 'intelligence is related to achievement' is too vague about the exact variables that will be used to measure intelligence and achievement. An improved hypothesis might be 'IQ is related to A level grades'.

By explicitly formulating the hypothesis prior to the study you can avoid fitting in a hypothesis that fits the data ('cooking the books'). Ignoring one's original predictions in favour of incidental findings is dangerous. The problem with such a strategy is that, if enough hypotheses are set after data collection, eventually the finding that emerges will be by chance and due to the manipulations of the variables.

In order to carry out an inferential statistical test on an experimental hypothesis it must be possible in principle for the predicted effects either to occur or not to occur. For example, the experimental hypothesis 'use of crutches will improve ability to walk' can be supported if the patients' overall mobility improves after using crutches. Or, the experimental hypothesis can be unsupported if the patients display no differences in mobility regardless of whether they have been given crutches or not. An experimental hypothesis is always tested against a null hypothesis, where a null hypothesis states that a researcher will not find the experimental results that they expected and that any results are due to chance fluctuations in performances rather than the effects of any variable.

Issues around research design

In considering the influence that research design will have on the inferential statistical test you choose, we will consider the number of conditions, the number of independent variables and the allocation of subjects to conditions. An experiment can have two or more conditions. An experiment may have two conditions if there is one experimental condition and one control condition. An experimental condition is a condition in which people are subjected to the independent variable while a control condition is a condition in which people are not subjected to the independent variable.

Example:
Experimental condition   *Control condition*
Pretest scores   Pretest scores
Treatment   No treatment
Post-test scores   Post-test scores

An experiment can have two experimental conditions. For example, if you were conducting a test into which set of instructions is easier to remember, short or long, the independent variable is instruction length, which has two levels (conditions): short and long. It is also possible to look at more than two levels of an independent variable. For example, short, medium and long instructions or short, medium and no instructions.

It is often the case that a particular variable may have one effect on people's behaviour in one situation and quite another effect in another situation. For example, one treatment might be better at improving mobility in children, while another treatment might be better at improving mobility in adults. This gives us two independent variables: age and treatment. You can design a two-by-two experiment to look at both of these variables (see Table 9.3).

In this design, subjects in both age groups would be given both treatments in order to see what effect treatment has on mobility scores and what effect age has on mobility scores. From the example in Table 9.3 you can see that both age and treatment are having a main effect because the total scores for A are less than those for B and the total scores for young subjects are higher than those for older subjects. There is also an interaction between age and treatment because young people do better on treatment A while older people do better on treatment B. It is possible to look at any number of variables, each with any number of conditions.

In considering the allocation of subjects to conditions you will need to check whether you have a different or same subject design. A different subject (unrelated) design is where you use different people for each experimental condition.

Table 9.3   A two-by-two experimental design

Age	Treatment		Totals
	A	B	
Young	10	6	16
Old	1	12	13
Totals	11	18	29

Example:

Subject	Treatment A	Subject	Treatment B
1	2	6	4
2	4	7	5
3	6	8	9
4	4	9	3
5	3	10	10

The advantage of a different subject design is that it can avoid the possibility of order effects which can affect performance. Where there are different people in each condition, the experience of one condition cannot be carried over to the other conditions. The disadvantage of a different subject design is that there may be individual differences in the way different subjects tackle the experimental task, and therefore performance may be affected by variables other than those manipulated by the experimenter.

A same subject (related) design is a design where you use the same subjects for all experimental conditions.

Example:

Subject	Treatment A	Treatment B
1	10	12
2	9	10
3	11	4
4	8	6
5	5	9

The main advantage of a same subject design is that using the same subjects for all experimental conditions can eliminate the problem of individual differences more effectively than random allocation of different subjects. Any individual peculiarities get equalized out over all the conditions. The disadvantages of using a same subject design are that it cannot be used when subjects have to be different and, in using the same people for each condition, their experiences of each condition can affect how they perform on the condition (order effects).

A matched subject design attempts to combine the advantages of both related and unrelated designs. The experimenter tries to match the subjects doing each experimental condition on as many factors as possible which seem important for a particular experiment. Such factors may be gender, age or ability. A matched subject design can be treated as a related design. For the purposes of the experiment, matched subjects are as near as possible to same subjects. The advantage of a matched subject design is that it eliminates individual differences between experimental conditions. The disadvantages of a matched subject design are that it is often impossible to find subjects who are matched on all relevant characteristics and one can never be sure that subjects are matched on the variables that are likely to affect performance.

**Issues around the
nature of data**

In considering the influence that the nature of your research data will
have on the inferential statistical test you choose, we will look at levels
of measurement and the distribution and variation of data. There are
four levels of measurement: nominal, ordinal, interval and ratio (see
also Chapter 7). Nominal data are numbers that are merely used to
classify objects, such as bus numbers. Nominal data also include
frequencies when you are counting how many people or things fall into
particular categories. For example, how many outpatients at hospital A
and B completed their course of treatment? Just as it does not make
much sense to carry out mathematical operations on bus numbers, it is
nonsensical to carry out mathematical operations on nominal data.

Ordinal data involve arranging data in order or rank, such as
preferences or social class measurements. However, the numbers are
not absolute and there is no guarantee that the distance between first
and second or good and medium is the same as the distance between
second and third or medium and bad. Therefore, adding, subtracting,
dividing or multiplying this kind of data does not make much sense.

Interval data involve arranging data in order, but there are equal
intervals between successive points on the scale. Examples include
temperature, IQ and year of birth. The interval scale has no absolute
zero, only a man-made zero such as 0°C. As there is no absolute zero
you can talk about subzero points. Mathematical operations can be
carried out on this kind of data.

Ratio data can be arranged in order, with equal intervals and an
absolute zero. For example, length, reaction times and number of
correct responses. The zero point on this scale literally means zero. It
does not make sense to talk about −4 inches or −10 kilograms.
Mathematical operations can be carried out on this kind of data.

Consideration of the distribution and variation of data centres on
understanding normal distribution and homogeneity of variance. There
are a number of frequency distribution shapes that occur commonly in
statistics. The most common is the normal distribution curve. This
curve is symmetrical and bell-shaped (see Figure 9.3). With a normal
distribution curve the mean, median and mode all have the same
value.

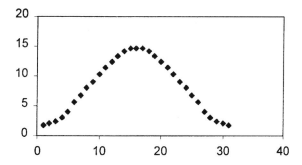

Figure 9.3   Normal distribution curve.

If the mean and standard deviation of a set of scores are known, then the researcher is able to predict what proportion of the population has scores within a certain range. This is because a fixed proportion of the population will fall within a certain score range, as long as those scores are normally distributed. Establishing whether your data has homogeneity of variance involves checking whether the variability (usually standard deviation) of scores in each condition is approximately the same.

Parametric and non-parametric tests

There are two kinds of inferential statistical tests: parametric and non-parametric. With a parametric test it is possible to calculate exact numerical scores which indicate the proportions of total variability in scores that are due to independent variables or unknown variables. Parametric tests are so called because various assumptions are made about the parameters of the data under consideration. Parametric tests assume that the data are either interval or ratio (since it is possible to carry out numerical calculations on the data, it is not sufficient simply to rank the data in order). They also assume that the scores are normally distributed, there is equal variance (or, alternatively, there need to be equal numbers in each group) and the subjects have been randomly selected. Parametric tests should only be used if these conditions are met. However, while the first condition is essential, the other three can be violated to some extent.

Non-parametric tests do not calculate exact numerical differences between scores; the tests only take into account whether certain scores are higher or lower than other scores. They do not make assumptions about the distribution or the variance of the data under consideration and can be used on nominal or ordinal data.

Parametric tests are more powerful and therefore more likely to pick up significant differences. They can also look at more than one independent variable. Conversely, non-parametric tests are less powerful and unable to look at more than one variable and can therefore ignore the complexities of human behaviour. However, they are easy and quick and able to look at trends in scores.

From your hypothesis:
1. Are you looking at differences or associations?

From your design:
2. Have you got the same, matched or different subject design?
3. How many conditions do you have?
4. How many variables are there?

From your data:
5. Is the data nominal, ordinal, interval or ratio?
6. Is the data normally distributed?
7. Is the variance in each condition similar?

Figure 9.4   Questions to consider when choosing a statistical test.

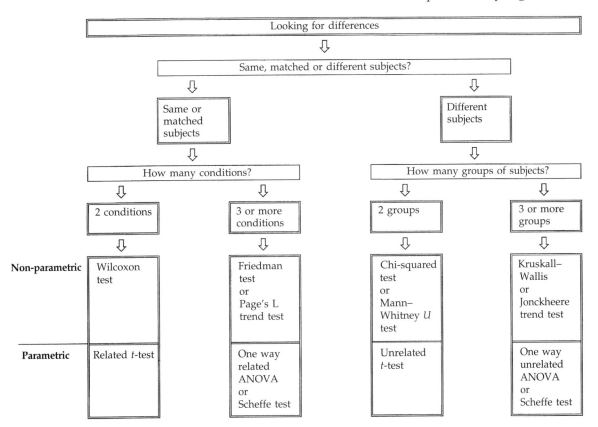

Figure 9.5   Statistical test decision flow chart when looking for differences.

Choosing the right inferential statistical test

Choosing the right statistical test involves asking a set of questions (see Figure 9.4). The process of asking these questions and making decisions about the answer will lead you down a path to a choice of one or two named statistical tests. Figure 9.5 outlines the decision flow chart when looking for differences (with just one independent variable). Figure 9.6 outlines the decision flow chart when looking for associations (see also Hicks, 1995 and McCall, 1996).

Different books and different computer packages may call statistical tests by slightly different names. For example, the *t*-test is a parametric test that can be used to test differences of one variable with two conditions. The *t*-test is sometimes called the Student's *t*-test. In addition there a two types of *t*-test, one for when your subjects are the same in both conditions (related *t*-test) and one for when the subjects are different in both conditions (unrelated or independent sample *t*-test).

Whilst different names for the same test can be confusing, you need to be absolutely sure you have chosen the right test. Sometimes, even though you have chosen the wrong test, it is possible for your data to fit the formulae and to calculate a result. But just because you manage

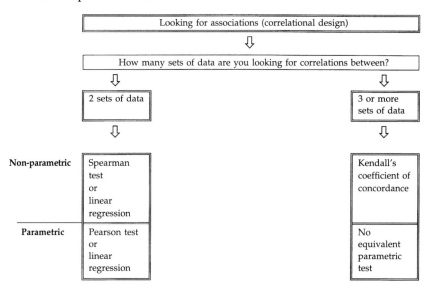

Figure 9.6   Statistical test decision flow chart when looking for associations.

to get a result out of a statistical test does not necessarily mean that you have chosen the right one. Even if you are planning on asking a computer to carry out a statistical analysis, you still need to tell it which test to conduct.

Understanding the results from a statistical test

In using inferential statistics to test experimental hypotheses, we are attempting to determine the acceptability of the hypothesis. A hypothesis is considered acceptable if the results are significantly different from those that would be produced by chance. With the example of before and after scores (see Table 9.4), 80% of the measurements show an improvement after treatment, while 20% of measurements worsened. A statistical test allows us to determine whether this 80:20 ratio is significantly different from a 50:50 ratio that we would expect by chance.

Table 9.4   Comparison of before and after scores

Before	After	Improved (+) or worsened (−)
5	7	+
8	5	−
10	11	+
7	10	+
13	15	+
6	7	+
12	9	−
13	17	+
17	19	+
12	15	+

The end result of running a statistical test is a number or test statistic. This test statistic is compared with values (critical values) in special statistical tables. Statistical tables provide a distribution of all the probabilities of experimental scores occurring by chance. If this probability (p) is small, less than or equal to 0.05 or 0.01, then the experimental hypothesis can be accepted. If the probability is larger than 0.05 or 0.01 then any apparent effect found in the data is probably due to chance and we can accept the null hypothesis. These probability values are called levels of significance.

If p is greater than (>) 0.05, the test statistic is not significant at the 5% level because there is a 95% probability of the results being due to chance. If p is less than (<) 0.05, the test statistic is significant at the 5% level because there is 95% probability of the results not being due to chance. The smaller the p value, the more significant the results are. A difference which is significant at the 1% level is more convincing evidence of a real difference than one which is significant at the 5% level.

For a hypothesis which predicts a difference only in one direction (one-tailed), there is a specific percentage probability that the difference might occur by chance. If a hypothesis makes a prediction that a difference might occur in either direction (two-tailed) then there is double the probability that such differences might occur by chance. There is the probability that the results might occur in one direction, plus the probability that the differences might occur in the other direction. Each statistical test has its own probability table. These are usually listed in the back of statistical textbooks such as Hick (1995) and McCall (1996).

Example: A study was conducted to compare the number of non-verbal behaviours that two physiotherapists displayed. A statistical test was conducted in order to test the hypothesis that one physiotherapist would display more verbal behaviours than the other would. A test statistic of 3.338 is produced. The relevant statistical tables reveal critical values at five levels of significance (see Table 9.5). In order to be significant at one of these levels the test statistic has to be equal to or larger than one of these critical values. Our test statistic of 3.338 is larger than the critical value for 10% but smaller than the critical value for 5%. Therefore, for a two-tailed hypothesis the test statistic is significant at the 10% level. However, since we made a one-tailed hypothesis, we need to halve the p value shown for a two-tailed hypothesis. Therefore for a one-tailed hypothesis, the test statistic is significant at the 5% level.

Table 9.5   Example of probability table for a two-tailed hypothesis

Levels of probability	0.10 (10%)	0.05 (5%)	0.02 (2%)	0.01 (1%)	0.001 (0.1%)
Critical Values	2.71	3.84	5.41	6.64	10.83

Manual and computer analysis of quantitative data

Unless you have a small amount of data, it is probably unwise to analyse your data by hand. Analysing large data sets by hand is time consuming, onerous and can lead to errors in calculation that may be difficult to detect. If you wish to analyse quantitative data by hand then you need to be sure that you know how to operate the formula in question.

A common computer package used to analyse quantitative data is the Statistical Package for Social Sciences (SPSS). SPSS allows you to store your data, perform statistical analyses and produce charts and graphs of results. Data are entered using a spreadsheet and the results of the analyses are displayed in a separate output window. The data, the output and the commands you have given SPSS can be saved independently for future sessions. The output tables can also be copied to a word processing application for inclusion in reports.

SPSS can handle different types of data. Questionnaire designers like SPSS because it does not insist on having numerical data. For example, it can handle textual data such as m for male and f for female. It can also handle numerically coded data such as 1 for occupational therapists, 2 for physiotherapist and 3 for doctor. What SPSS does require you to do is to define your data before you start by assigning 'value labels' (see Chapter 10 for an example).

Key points

1. The main steps in analysing qualitative data are preparing, analysing and interpreting.
2. Indexing, diagrams and charts are methods of manually analysing qualitative data.
3. Text retrieval, description and theory building are three types of computer analysis that can be used with qualitative data.
4. Quantitative data can be analysed using descriptive or inferential statistics.
5. The mean, median and mode are three measures of central tendency.
6. The range and standard deviation are two measures of dispersion.
7. The number of conditions and independent variables and using the same or different subjects will influence the choice of statistical test.
8. Levels of measurement and distribution of data influence the choice of statistical test.
9. Statistical tests can be parametric or non-parametric.
10. We need to make sure we have chosen the right statistical test.
11. Computer analysis of quantitative data is probably easier than manual analysis for large data sets.
12. A common computer analysis package is SPSS.

References

Bryman, A. and Burgess, R.G. (1994). *Analysing Qualitative Data*. Routledge.
Hicks, C. (1995). *Research for Physiotherapists*. Churchill Livingstone.
Mason, J. (1996). *Qualitative Researching*. Sage Publications.
McCall, J. (1996). *Statistics: A Guide for Therapists*. Butterworth-Heinemann.

Seale, J. (1993). *Microcomputers in adult special education: the management of innovation*. PhD Thesis (2 volumes), Keele University.

Tesch, R. (1990). *Qualitative Research: Analysis Types and Software Tools*. Falmer.

Complementary reading

Coffey, A. and Atkinson, P. (1996). *Making Sense of Qualitative Data. Complementary Research Strategies*. Sage Publications. Chapter 2: Concepts and coding.

French, S. (1993). *Practical Research: A Guide for Therapists*. Butterworth-Heinemann. Chapter 11: Basic statistical concepts.

Mason, J. (1994). Linking qualitative and quantitative data analysis. In *Analysing Qualitative Data*. (A. Bryman and R.G. Burgess, eds), pp. 89–110. Routledge.

Miles, M.B. and Huberman, A.M. (1994). *Qualitative Data Analysis: An Expanded Sourcebook*. Sage Publications.

10 **Analysis of questionnaires**

Getting started

In Chapter 4 we covered issues surrounding the design of questionnaires. When it comes to thinking about questionnaire analysis several points need to be noted. When designing a questionnaire it is advisable to plan how you are going to analyse the data before you start distributing your questionnaires. Part of this planning will involve deciding whether you want to analyse the data manually or by computer. This decision may be influenced by how computer literate you feel, how many completed questionnaires you hope to get and the nature of the questions asked. Usually we would advise people not to use a lack of computer literacy as an excuse for avoiding using a computer for data analysis. There are some good manuals around, your supervisor may be able to help you or your school or department may run introductory courses. However, it will take some time to learn to use a computer package, code the data and label the variables. We would advise you to incorporate this time into your project time-scale.

If you are expecting fewer than 20 questionnaires back or have some open questions then it may be preferable to analyse the data by hand. Realistically, it is likely that most questionnaire studies will involve open and closed questions, thus requiring some manual and some computerized analysis. This chapter will demonstrate some useful analysis techniques using a sample questionnaire that incorporates both open and closed questions.

Sample questionnaire

The questionnaire that we are going to use in this chapter (see Figure 10.1) was designed to provide evaluative data for a multimedia teaching package that had been designed for use with occupational therapy students and clinicians (Seale, 1997). Specifically, the researcher who used this questionnaire wanted to investigate whether previous IT experience had any influence on how easy respondents found the package to use. Before we launch into how we might analyse the questionnaire, take five minutes to read it. Note the instructions, the range of question types used and the structuring of the questionnaire from background information to personal opinions.

Analysis choices

It would be possible to use a computer package to analyse the open questions in this questionnaire. For example, McComas *et al.* (1995) used 'Ethnograph' to analyse responses to four open questions in a

Computer Applications in Therapy: Evaluation of a multimedia teaching package
In order to evaluate the educational effectiveness of the multimedia package called Computer Applications in Therapy (CAT) I am trying to gain as much information as possible regarding how easy the package is to use and what influence previous IT experience has on ease of use. It would be really helpful if you could take 10 minutes to complete this questionnaire. Your constructive comments are welcomed, whether positive or negative. For the purposes of this research, confidential details such as name are not required; therefore complete anonymity is assured.

Please read each question carefully and respond as directed.

SECTION 1: BACKGROUND INFORMATION
AND PREVIOUS EXPERIENCE

1. Are you are student or a clinician? Please tick the appropriate box.

   Student ☐   Clinician ☐

2a. Have you used a Windows package before? Please tick the appropriate box.

   YES ☐   NO ☐

2b. If you have ticked the YES box, how would you rate yourself as a Windows user? Please tick the appropriate box.

   I have basic Windows skills ☐

   I have intermediate Windows skills ☐

   I have expert Windows skills ☐

3a. Have you used the World Wide Web (WWW) before? Please tick the appropriate box.

   YES ☐   NO ☐

3b. If you have ticked the YES box, how would you rate yourself as a WWW user? Please tick the appropriate box.

   Basic WWW skills ☐

   Intermediate WWW skills ☐

   Expert WWW skills ☐

4. Have you used a multimedia teaching package such as CAT before? Please tick the appropriate box.

   YES ☐   NO ☐

4b. If you have ticked the YES box please give a brief description of the package here:

5a. Have you used a computer as a therapeutic tool with clients?

   YES ☐   NO ☐

5b. If you have ticked the YES box please give a brief description of use here:

SECTION 2: CAT AND EASE OF USE

Please read the statements below and ring the response that is closest to your view or opinion.
(1 = strongly disagree, 5 = strongly agree.)

It was clear what options were available to me.	1 2 3 4 5
The screens were easy to read.	1 2 3 4 5
The content of the package was at the wrong level for me.	1 2 3 4 5
I frequently got disorientated within the package.	1 2 3 4 5
I was able to create a conceptual map of the resource material.	1 2 3 4 5
It was easy to move between the case histories and the resource material.	1 2 3 4 5
I found it difficult to develop a search strategy.	1 2 3 4 5

Please feel free to write any comments you may have regarding how easy the CAT package was to use and any possible influence your previous IT experience had on you use of the package.

Figure 10.1   Sample questionnaire.

questionnaire that was designed to explore how physiotherapists deal with inappropriate patient sexual behaviour. An example of one of the open questions included in the questionnaire was: 'Do you have any comments to make about how you learned to deal with inappropriate patient sexual behaviour?'. For this study 152 questionnaires were returned. With 608 open responses to analyse it is not surprising that these researchers chose to use a computer package. The researchers used an initial review of the data to devise a preliminary conceptual framework. This framework identified themes for each question and operational definitions. The operational definitions were used to code the transcriptions. The themes were then grouped and linked together to identify some overarching concepts. For example, the themes of changing own behaviour, discussing with client and disclosing formed a concept called 'coping strategies'.

Let's assume that with our sample questionnaire only 30 completed questionnaires were returned. With such a small number of question-naires it is probably not worth analysing the open responses by computer. It would also be possible to analyse the closed questions by hand. This would probably involve simple frequencies on the most part, which could be recorded in some kind of table (see Table 10.1).

While working frequencies out by hand is often useful for a first or overall impression of the data, it does not allow a more in-depth investigation to occur. For example, from this table we do not know how many students said they could use a Windows package, or how many basic Windows users strongly disagreed that the options were clear. This kind of analysis is called cross-tabulation, which essentially involves cross-referencing responses to one question to responses to

Table 10.1 Summarizing closed questions by hand

Question	Frequencies				
Are you are student or a clinician?	Student ✓✓✓✓✓ ✓✓✓✓✓ ✓✓✓✓✓ ✓✓✓✓✓	Clinician ✓✓✓✓✓✓ ✓✓✓✓			
Have you used a Windows package before?	Yes ✓✓✓✓✓ ✓✓✓✓✓ ✓✓✓✓✓ ✓✓✓✓✓	No ✓✓✓✓✓			
How would you rate yourself as a Windows user?	Basic ✓✓✓✓✓ ✓✓✓✓✓ ✓	Intermediate ✓✓✓✓✓✓✓ ✓	Expert ✓✓		
Ratings for statement 1: It was clear what options were available to me.	Strongly agree ✓✓✓✓✓ ✓✓✓✓✓ ✓✓✓✓✓ ✓✓✓✓	Agree ✓✓✓✓✓✓ ✓✓✓✓	Neutral ✓✓✓✓✓ ✓	Disagree	Strongly disagree

another question. Such analysis is probably easier to do using a computer package. This chapter will now go on to outline how you might use a statistical package such as SPSS to code and analyse responses to closed questions.

Computerized analysis of closed questions

In Chapter 9 we discussed how SPSS is particularly useful because it can handle textual and numerical data. In order to enable SPSS to handle such different types of data we are required to define our data by assigning value and variable labels. Value labels are the codes that you give to your data such as 1 for yes and 2 for no. Variable labels are the codes or names you give to each question answer. When you enter data using the data editor, each row corresponds to each respondent or subject in the study and each column corresponds to each variable or question answer. SPSS automatically names each variable or column for you, for example 'var00001' for column 1. Such names are not particularly informative. You can rename these variables to something more meaningful. SPSS allows you to give each variable a code up to eight characters long (e.g. STUDCLIN) and a label which gives more information about what the code actually means (e.g. student or clinician). If we turn our attention back to the sample questionnaire, before we can use SPSS to analyse responses to the closed questions we need to create a coding grid (see Table 10.2).

From Table 10.2 you can see that the researcher has coded the variables so that they are all numeric with just one character. It is possible that a different researcher would code the same data in a different way. For example, the variable STUDCLIN could be a string variable with labels c for clinician and s for student. Whichever way a researcher decides to code their data they need to make sure that it is clearly labelled and defined, otherwise the results that SPSS produces will make little sense.

Once you have coded and defined your data, the laborious task of data entry awaits! Researchers often pay other people to do the data entry task, as it is rather time consuming. Whether you pay someone or do it yourself beware that errors can occur. Table 10.3 shows how the SPSS data sheet for a sample questionnaire might look once you have finished data entry. As this coding grid involves data from just 10 respondents it is possible to see potential patterns. For example, from columns 3 and 4 we can see, that while most people have used Windows, the majority are rating themselves as a 1 (basic) in terms of ability to use Windows. From column 8 we can see from the large number of 2s (no) that the majority of respondents have not used the computer as a therapeutic tool with clients. If your data set is quite large then an initial inspection of the coding grid is unlikely to yield obvious patterns. SPSS, however, can quite quickly reveal patterns that may need further exploration through the use of descriptive statistics.

Descriptive statistics

There are a number of descriptive analyses that SPSS can conduct. With our sample data set we can ask SPSS to produce frequency tables

Table 10.2   Example of SPSS coding grid

Variable name	Question/variable label	Value labels
STUDCLIN	Are you are student or a clinician?	Student = 1 Clinician = 2 Missing data = 9
USEDWIN	Have you used a Windows package before?	Yes = 1 No = 2 Missing data = 9
WINSKILL	How would you rate yourself as a Windows user?	Basic = 1 Intermediate = 2 Expert = 3 Missing data = 9
USEDWWW	Have you used the World Wide Web?	Yes = 1 No = 2 Missing data = 9
WWWSKILL	How would you rate yourself as a World Wide Web user?	Basic = 1 Intermediate = 2 Expert = 3 Missing data = 9
MMTP	Have you used a multimedia teaching package such as CAT before?	Yes = 1 No = 2 Missing data = 9
COMPTHER	Have you used a computer as a therapeutic tool with clients?	Yes = 1 No = 2 Missing data = 9
STATE1–STATE7	Opinion statements	Strongly disagree = 1 Disagree = 2 Neutral = 3 Agree = 4 Strongly agree = 5 Missing data = 9

Table 10.3   Sample SPSS data table

Id	stud clin	used win	win skill	used www	www skill	mmtp	comp ther	state1	state2
1	1	1	1	1	1	2	2	4	5
2	1	1	1	1	1	2	2	4	5
3	1	1	1	1	1	2	2	4	5
4	2	1	1	1	1	2	2	4	4
5	1	1	2	1	2	1	2	4	5
6	2	1	1	1	1	1	2	5	5
7	1	1	1	1	1	2	2	4	4
8	1	1	2	2	9	1	1	4	4
9	1	1	1	1	2	2	2	4	4
10	2	1	1	2	9	2	1	4	4

Table 10.4 Extract from SPSS syntax file

```
FREQUENCIES
VARIABLES = state1 state2 state3 state4 state5 state6 state7
/STATISTICS = STDDEV RANGE MEAN MEDIAN MODE.
CROSSTABS
/TABLES = wwwskill BY state1 state2 state3 state4 state5 state6 state7
/FORMAT = AVALUE NOINDEX BOX LABELS TABLES
/CELLS = COUNT .
GRAPH
/BAR(GROUPED) = COUNT BY state2 BY winskill
/MISSING = REPORT.
```

that display the number of times each code (category of the variable) occurs. In addition we can ask for all the measurements of central tendency and dispersion to be reported. Provided we specify which variables (question answers) we are interested in we can also ask SPSS to run a cross-tabulation. Finally, SPSS can produce charts and graphs of specified variables of interest. Table 10.4 shows an extract from an SPSS syntax file that asks SPSS to conduct the following operations:

1. Calculate frequencies for the variables state1 to state7.
2. Calculate the standard deviation, range, mean, median and mode for the variables state1 to state7.
3. Conduct a cross-tabulation for the variable wwwskill by variables state1 to state7.
4. Plot a graph delineating how people of different Windows skills responded to statement 2.
5. Report all missing cases.

SPSS outputs results from requested analyses into a separate file. This file can be saved or printed. Examples of descriptive results produced by SPSS are shown in Tables 10.5 and 10.6 and Figure 10.2. They give you a feel for how results may be presented and also remind us of how important it is for us to label and define variables. From the example in Table 10.5, we can see that by giving a variable label to the variable STATE2 we are easily reminded what the statement was that people are responding to. By giving value labels we can easily and quickly make sense of the data. For example, we can see that 15 people agreed to the statement that the screens were easy to read. Without a value label all we would know is that 15 people responded with a '4'.

From the example in Table 10.5 we can also see that the majority of responses to the question 'were the screens easy to read' were positive. The small standard deviation and the range of 2 indicate that there was not a great variation in the responses. However, given that the numbers are not absolute numbers but codes, it probably makes more sense to use the range as an indicator of variation. All the averages (mean, median and mode) are the same, indicating that that average

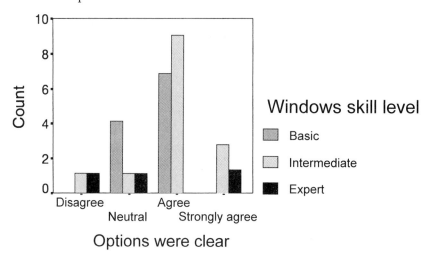

Figure 10.2 Graph to show how people of different Windows skills responded to statement 2.

Table 10.5 SPSS calculation of frequencies for statement 2

STATE2: screens easy to read

Value label	Value	Frequency	Per cent	Valid per cent	Cum. per cent
Neutral	3	3	10.0	10.0	10.0
Agree	4	15	50.0	50.0	60.0
Strongly agree	5	12	40.0	40.0	100.0
Total		30	100.0	100.0	

Mean	4.300	Median	4.000	Mode	4.000
SD	0.651	Range	2.000		
Valid cases	30	Missing cases	0		

response to the question was 4 (agree). However, given the nature of the data, it probably makes more sense to focus on the mode and conclude that the most common (frequent) response was to agree to the statement.

An inspection of the analysis in Table 10.6 reveals that there were more 'basic' World Wide Web (WWW) users than 'intermediate' and 'expert'; most people either agreed or disagreed with statement 1 and more 'basic' World Wide Web users agreed than disagreed with the statement. SPSS also tells us what percentage of the total group each score accounts for. So, for example, we know that half (50%) of the respondents were basic WWW users. It is difficult to make much of this cross-tabulation since there were so few intermediate or expert users.

Table 10.6   SPSS cross-tabulation of WWWSKILL (how would you rate yourself as a www user?) by STATE1 (options were clear)

WWWSKILL	STATE1: Disagree	Neutral	Agree	Strongly agree	Row total
	2	3	4	5	
Basic 1	1		11	3	15 50.0
Intermediate 2		1		1	2 6.7
Expert 3		1			1 3.3
Missing 9	1	5	6		12 40.0
Column total	2 6.7	7 23.3	17 56.7	4 13.3	30 100.0

Number of missing observations: 0

The results from the graph in Figure 10.2 demonstrate another cross-tabulation. From this graph we can see that 'intermediate' and 'expert' Windows users tended to use the whole range of responses. The majority of 'basic' and 'intermediate' users agreed that the options were clear. Opinion seems to be divided amongst the 'expert' users.

Inferential statistics

SPSS can conduct a number of non-parametric and parametric inferential statistical analyses. Unfortunately, SPSS cannot tell you which is the right test to choose! So be clear which independent variables you want to test and whether the dependent variables that measure the independent variables will necessitate a parametric or non-parametric test. Whilst SPSS takes a lot of the mathematical work out of using statistical tests it does not produce a nice statement saying 'your results are significant at the $n\%$ level'. You will need to be able to interpret the significance of the results.

If we wanted to test whether ratings on statement 3 were significantly different for those who had used computers as a therapeutic tool compared to those who had not we could run an inferential statistical test. The ratings (1–5) are probably indicative of ordinal data, which suggests a non-parametric test. The two groups are independent in that those who have used a computer as a therapeutic tool cannot also be in the group who have not used the computer as a therapeutic tool. These assumptions would lead us to choose a Mann–Whitney test (see Hicks, 1995 and McCall, 1996).

The first thing you will notice from the example in Table 10.7 is that two tests have been run: the Mann–Whitney and the Wilcoxon. For the

Table 10.7   SPSS results for a Mann–Whitney test

Mann-Whitney U–Wilcoxon rank sum W test

STATE3: content at wrong level by COMPTHER: have you used a computer as a therapeutic tool?

Mean rank	Cases
13.77	11 COMPTHER = 1 Yes
16.50	19 COMPTHER = 2 No

Total = 30

	Exact:			Corrected for ties:	
U	W	Two-tailed p		Z	Two-tailed p
85.5	151.5	0.4197		−0.8889	0.3741

Mann–Whitney you will need to focus on test statistic U. The second thing to note is that SPSS has run a two-tailed test. An inspection of a statistical book will reveal that in order to be significant U has to be equal to or less than the critical value. SPSS does not tell you what the critical value is. What it does tell you is that the p value is 0.4197. This means that the results are significant at the 41% level. In other words, there is a 59% probably that any difference between the two groups is due to chance. These results are therefore highly insignificant.

Manual analysis of open questions

At the end of the questionnaire there is an open question which asks respondents to discuss how easy the package was to use and the

Table 10.8   Raw data for open question regarding how easy the package was to use

Positive:
1. I thought the CAT package was a helpful and interesting method of finding out information. It kept me interested and allowed me to look into more detail at specific areas of the subject that interested me.
2. Having accessed CAT once, the ease of use has encouraged me to return to it for both research information and for interest.
3. Took a little while to get to grips with how to access the required information, but once accessed – brilliant – very useful, clear!
4. I found it quite easy and information helpful.

Negative:
1. Overall very easy to use, however it was hard to know where to start your research and you always wanted to know whether you'd extracted all relevant knowledge.
2. I felt I needed to be able to jot down ? information as it came up, as otherwise I was unsure how to get back and retrieve it.
3. With the case study Malcolm I was not able to find relevant information that I had thought was pertinent to the case. I was left wondering what to do and if I had missed all the information somewhere.

Table 10.9 Raw data for influence of previous IT experience

Positive:
1. It (CAT) was easy to use as I have a very basic understanding of computers.
2. Previous IT experience had some advantage probably in confidence levels and therefore confidence to explore and not afraid of 'getting it wrong'.
3. Having used a computer before did help me with using the CAT package.
4. Although I have little experience of IT I do feel that I would be inclined to use it in my free time. It looks very interesting.
5. I was pleasantly surprised how easy it was to use considering my limited computer experience.
6. By knowing how to enlarge screens and viewing different pages, it was easier to navigate myself through the files. May be more complicated for someone with few computing skills.

Negative:
1. It wasn't hard to use although I'm not very good (or used) with computers – I feel I didn't use it to its maximum potential because of this.
2. My lack of experience made it quite difficult to find my way around the package. It was reasonably easy to use with practice.
3. Because of my previous experience I wandered round rather than pursuing the subject of Malcolm at all times.

possible influence that previous IT experience had on their use of the package. A manual analysis of these responses will need to begin by transcribing all the responses. This first analysis can be broken down by listing all the responses to 'how easy was the package to use' (see Table 10.8) and all the responses regarding the possible influence of previous IT experience (see Table 10.9). At this stage it may also be possible to group responses into positive and negative statements. There may be statements that do not fall into these two categories which need to be recorded in a separate category. However, we have still got raw data that need summarizing. This may be achieved by examining the statements and trying to identify themes. For example, an examination of the statements regarding how easy the package was to use allows us to identify four themes: finding the package interesting, having access to information, quality of information and ability to access information. An examination of the statements regarding the influence of previous IT experience reveals a focus on navigation and exploration (see Table 10.10).

Analysis of open responses can be problematic. Some people's written responses are difficult to read or not in complete English. Sometimes we have to assume that what someone has written is not actually what they wanted to say. For example, did the person who wrote the comment 'liked the idea of following skills' mean to say they liked the idea of 'following links'? Perhaps the biggest problem with trying to draw up categories is that it can be difficult to place some statements into any of your identified categories. Finally, differing researchers may place the same statement in different

Table 10.10 Identifying themes

Ease of use:

	Themes	Examples
Positive opinions	Finding the package interesting. Access to information.	It kept me interested. It was an interesting and helpful method of finding out information.
Negative opinions	Quality of information (missing or not relevant).	I was left wondering if I had missed all the information somewhere.
	Ability to access information.	I was unsure how to get back and retrieve it.

Influence of previous IT skills:

Themes	Categories	Examples
Positive opinions	Exploration/navigation	Confidence to explore. It was easier to navigate.
Negative opinions	Exploration/navigation	Difficult to find my way around. I wandered rather than pursued.

categories. For a large study it may be useful to employ a number of researchers who can verify interpretation given to open responses.

Key points

1. Careful planning is needed when deciding how to analyse questionnaires.
2. A computer package such as SPSS can provide descriptive and inferential analysis of data from closed questions.
3. You can manually reduce raw data from open questions into themes and categories.

References

Hicks, C. (1995). *Research for Physiotherapists*. Churchill Livingstone.
McCall, J. (1996). *Statistics: A Guide for Therapists*. Butterworth-Heinemann.
McComas, J., Kaplan, D. and Giacomin, C. (1995). Inappropriate patient sexual behaviour in physiotherapy practice: a qualitative analysis of questionnaire comments. *Physiotherapy Canada*, **47**, 127–133.
Seale, J. (1997). *The influence of previous IT skills on the use of a resource based occupational therapy multimedia teaching package*. Paper presented to the Learning Technology in Medical Education Conference, Bristol.

Complementary reading

Couchman, W. and Dawson, J. (1995). *Nursing and Healthcare Research*. Scutari Press. Chapter 7: Surveys.

11 Analysis of interviews

Approaches to analysing interview data

Chapter 5 looked at interviews as a research method and considered different types of interview. This chapter looks in more depth at the analysis of the qualitative data obtained from interviews, which Clark (1997) considers to be one of the most widely used techniques in the 'qualitative research toolkit'. The very formalized data from structured interviews is analysed similarly to questionnaire data and is addressed in Chapter 10. This chapter will look at what you do with all the qualitative data obtained from semi-structured and unstructured interviews. This data will offer a rich combination of perspective, experience and feeling that needs to be considered sensitively and thoroughly to reflect the true meanings of the participants.

Just as there are many and varied qualitative research methodologies and approaches, so there are many methods of analysis, often confounding in their complexity and terminology. Three types of qualitative analysis based on transcripts of interview data are discussed here: content analysis, thematic analysis and grounded theory analysis. Other analysis methods include conversation analysis, narrative analysis and discourse analysis (Payne, 1997).

Content analysis is the most basic of the interview data analyses. It is often used in patient satisfaction research and where researchers are exploring fact and experience. After reading the transcripts, the researcher codes the information into basic themes, relating directly to the questions asked or topics explored. This type of basic analysis is largely descriptive rather than analytical, the final report being based on the emergent themes.

Thematic analysis is used for more exploratory work, being more theoretical and analytical than content analysis. Analysis starts with the reading of the transcripts and coding of issues arising, which are organized into more general themes. As the data collection and analysis progresses, themes are identified and clarified. The research topic informs these themes and the discipline and academic interest of the researcher also plays a part. Emergent themes are further analysed, for example, by relating them to existing theory or creating a typology of attitudes or experiences. The final report is then based on these themes.

Grounded theory analysis is a more rigorous type of qualitative analysis. Transcripts are read and each few lines coded into issues that are then organized into conceptual categories. This process continues until the categories are saturated (i.e. no new data emerges) and it is possible to define the categories in terms of their limits and boundaries. This process involves the development and integration of new categories as the analysis progresses. These categories are then consolidated to develop a theory about the topic under investigation. This theory is then tested through more interviews for confirmation or modification and to test its limits. The final report is written on the basis of the theory that has been developed. The grounded theory approach is extremely rigorous and time consuming and is not feasible within the relatively short time-scale of an undergraduate project. Content and thematic analysis are the more common methods used.

Each of these three methods uses similar processes to identify the issues that arise. Data analysis begins immediately so that findings can inform subsequent interviews to 'improve the research process' (Glaser and Strauss, 1967; Maykut and Morehouse, 1994; Bowling, 1997). Transcripts are examined for the recurrence of themes within each interview and between interviewees. Key themes or categories are noted or developed. The results of the research may be presented in different ways. One commonly used method of presentation is the identification and description of the themes that have arisen (or, in grounded theory approach, by setting out the developed theories). These are then illustrated with quotes encapsulating the essence of the views of all participants or their range of opinions. The results may also give some indication as to the frequency of theme recurrence and whether different subgroups within the cohort expressed similar or disparate views (Seale, 1994).

Data preparation

Data from semi-structured and unstructured interviews can be collected in different ways (see Chapter 5). Usual methods are tape recordings and field notes. Before any analysis can take place the data must first be prepared. Field notes should be typed up as soon as possible after the interview. Robson (1993) warns of the dangers of losing valuable data if you return to it several months after the interview, simply because you can no longer remember how to translate your scribbled notes and abbreviations. As you type up the notes you are already starting to formulate some themes or categories from the data. Note them down. It does not matter how many you identify, as these can be refined as necessary at a later date.

Tape recordings can be prepared in several different ways according to the depth of analysis required. The first way does not require full transcription but does involve listening to the tape several times over to pick out themes. Ensure that the tape reel counter is set to zero at the start of the tape and note the reel count of each emerging theme. It is sensible to ask a colleague to listen to the tapes and identify the themes that emerge for them. In this way you can verify the validity of the themes. Do remember that you have assured interviewees of confidentiality so do ensure that your colleague cannot identify the voice on tape and reiterate the confidential nature of the process.

Noting down the reel count of relevant quotes enables you to find them easily and transcribe them to illustrate the emergent themes in the final report.

Full transcription is a time-consuming and often expensive process but is necessary if you wish to conduct a thorough and rigorous analysis. It also acts as another safeguard in the verification of themes by another person, as there is no possibility of them hearing and recognizing the voice of the interviewee.

The researcher can assist the transcriber by identifying the voices on the tape. Again, because of issues of confidentiality it is not always appropriate to give actual names (although this is difficult if people refer to each other by name on the tape). Simply clarifying the voices of interviewer and interviewee can be very helpful. Early on in the tape this is usually self-evident as the interviewer is asking the questions, but in tape recordings of focus groups it is difficult for transcribers to be absolutely sure who is speaking. The focus group facilitator and observer will need to assist in the identification process where this is necessary. Real names should not appear on the transcribed text.

Data analysis will be facilitated if transcription and field notes are typed double-spaced and any hard copies made on one side of the paper only. Leave wide margins to allow for coding.

Analysing the data

As already indicated, data is analysed by careful reading and rereading of transcripts or notes (or listening to tapes) and identifying themes. It is necessary to code themes on each transcript so that they can be compared with themes arising from other interviews. In practice there are many ways of doing this either by hand or using the computer. It is perfectly feasible to analyse small data sets by hand; however, even small data sets have a nasty habit of growing exponentially, so it is worth becoming familiar with a suitable software package if possible. Every researcher develops their own favourite method. If analysing data by hand make several photocopies of your scripts before you begin so that you can scribble on them or cut them up without damaging the original (Maykut and Morehouse, 1994). Ensure that you keep the original for reference and a pristine unmarked copy to give a colleague for validation. Several methods of coding and grouping data are described below.

1. Scribble key words and themes in the margins and consolidate once you have analysed all the scripts.
2. Use different coloured highlighter pens to identify different themes. Use a colour key to aid identification.
3. Use a filing card for each theme, then cut out and stick on to the cards the bits of text that relate to that theme. Remember to identify each cutting so that you can find them again in the full text. Maykut and Morehouse (1994) suggest that each transcript or page of field notes be coded to allow easy reference. They suggest that

each page is numbered, each interviewee is coded with the first letter of their name, and the type of data is coded, again by its first letter. Thus T/M-5 indicates that this cutting comes from page 5 (5) of a transcript (T) of an interview with Maria (M). Similarly, FN/P1-7 denotes page 7 of field notes (FN) of focus group 1 held with physiotherapists (P1). Ensure that you keep a key to the coding in your project journal or notes for later reference. It is important to be able to find themes again in scripts so that they can be refined and suitable quotes identified to illustrate the themes. The cards can be shuffled easily into more comprehensive categories or subcategories as the analysis progresses and more scripts are coded, allowing for a natural evolution of the final themes.

4. A more visual method is to type the script in large font and then, after coding sections with an identifier, cut them up and paste them on to large sheets of paper according to theme. These can then be fixed up on a large wall, allowing a great deal of data to be seen at one time for sorting into the most appropriate final themes. The authors have used the alternative method of spreading these sheets over the floor but recommend from experience that, if doing this at home, young children and pet cats are excluded from the room!

5. For easy identification and to prevent physically cutting up the scripts, use different coloured sticky dots on the scripts to cross-reference themes where more than one arises on each sheet. Remember to keep a key to the colours.

6. Data can also be categorized using the computer. Chapter 9 looks at some of the specialist software packages that can be used. It is also possible to use a simple word processing package, making use of the search or find facility to identify key words and phrases as a basis of themes and the cut and paste and notepad facilities to group themes and quotes. Using a computer window based environment allows for the easy movement of small amounts of data between files. The authors suggest purpose-built packages such as Nud.IST and Ethnograph for larger data sets (see Richards and Richards, 1994).

Example of content analysis

The hypothetical example in Figure 11.1 examines the possible themes that arise during analysis of a transcript of an interview with an elderly person talking about her experiences of a day hospital. Key words are noted in the margins and then developed into themes as the analysis progresses. In this example the researcher is simply looking for themes that relate directly to the interviewer's questions. The interviews sought only to gain information about fact and experience and the resultant data are most appropriately analysed in this way.

Although the first reading identifies many topics, further reading and comparison with other interviews will refine the themes. It is vital to look back at the research question to ensure that the data answer

I *is the interviewer* **Mrs W** *is the interviewee*	
	I: *What happens here at the day hospital?*
transport *coffee break* *'the girls'* *toilet* *physio*	**Mrs W:** Well, we get here on the transport and have a cup of coffee when we arrive. The girls are very good and take me to the toilet because we're all a bit desperate by then. Julie comes and gets me for my physio. I do some exercises and walk in the bars.
OT	**I:** *Do you have any other treatment?*
friends *frequency* *nursing treatment* *doctor*	**Mrs W:** I do some arm and hand exercises with the OTs. I talk to my friend, but she only comes on Thursdays and I'm here Mondays too. On Mondays the nurse gives me a bath and looks at my leg. She changes the dressing if it's sore and then I see the doctor sometimes too.
	I: *Are you aware of any other treatments available at the day hospital?*
'feet treatment' *waiting list* *food* *'the girls'*	**Mrs W:** You can have your feet done I think but there's a bit of a waiting list. We get lunch and have a bit of a rest afterwards. The food is quite good considering it's hospital food. There's not much of a choice and Dolly says it's too stodgy for her but I don't complain. These girls are doing their best. They are lovely girls. I don't think they get paid enough to look after us.
length of treatment	**I:** *How long have you been coming to the day hospital?*
Social Services *worries/concerns*	**Mrs W:** About . . . about a month. My doctor says I'll be here for a few weeks then he's going to get someone from the Social to help me out at home. I don't know what they do. I want someone to clean my place up a bit and help me in the bath. I don't know what will happen about my legs when I finish here. Who will change my dressings?

Figure 11.1 Content analysis of an interview transcript.

the question. When all the data have been analysed the resultant themes in this research are identified as:

1. Accessing the day hospital.
2. Uptake of health care services.
3. Perceived value of health care services.
4. Views on the day hospital environment and ancillary services.

5. Clients' perception of the outcome of day hospital attendance.
6. Clients' worries and concerns.

Theme 1: Secret fears
Children whose parents have MS can have secret feelings about it that they do not tell their parents. Sometimes without realizing it they can feel afraid.

'If I don't help Mummy her MS will get worse.'

'Unless I keep kicking my legs will stop working like Dad's.'

'If I feel dizzy or trip I think I've got MS.'

Theme 2: Children can feel responsible for the life and death of their parents
Sometimes children want their parents to get better so much they believe:

'If only I loved him properly he would get better.'

'I must be a very bad person because I cannot love Mum enough to make her better.'

'I must have done something wrong cos I prayed to God to make Mum better but now she uses a stick.'

Taken from Segal (undated) *Emotional Reactions to MS.*

Figure 11.2   Thematic analysis of an interview script.

Example of thematic analysis

The example in Figure 11.2 illustrates how themes have been identified from the interviews rather than set out in answer to specific questions. It looks at some of the responses of children being interviewed about their experiences of having a parent with multiple sclerosis. The first identified theme is 'secret fears'. Obviously these children were not asked, 'What are your secret fears relating to your mum or dad's MS?'. Rather, children were encouraged to explore their feelings about their family and personal circumstances and the researcher then drew out the commonly recurring themes from the entire interviews. The report, designed as an information booklet for parents with multiple sclerosis, sets out the various themes that arose and illustrates them with actual quotes from the participating children. It can be seen that this is a powerful way of presenting sensitive findings.

Example of grounded theory analysis

Oliver (1995) explored the counsellor's perspective of counselling disabled people using interviews and a grounded theory approach. She hoped that a central theme would emerge from the data which would enable a model or theory to be developed. Oliver describes how the data were broken down into manageable chunks following Strauss and Corbin's methodology (1990) in the two stages of open coding and axial coding. Open coding involved reading the scripts fully to get a feel for the data before breaking them down into the smallest sections that could stand alone. This resulted in 300 items for categorization.

The categories were created by 'starting with one item and finding the focus of what was being said in order to create a category'. Axial coding was then used to develop the paradigm model from the seven main categories found at open coding, exploring 'the properties and dimensions of each' to identify relationships. Oliver discusses the findings and identifies four points to her emerging theory:

1. Disabled people cannot be treated as a homogeneous group.
2. Disabled people need access to counselling that meets their specific needs.
3. Counselling should be flexible and aim to enable disabled people to empower themselves.
4. There are counsellors who are struggling to develop this approach.

Oliver does not feel that she can fully develop her theories, as her project was only able to look at one perspective. She notes that the client perspective needs inclusion to tell the full story.

Presenting analysed data

Once the data have been analysed, consideration needs to be given to their presentation in the final report. It is usual to set out the themes that have been identified, discuss the range of views that illustrate those themes and back them up using actual quotes. It may be possible to give some indication of how many interviewees identified the theme as important and illustrate this under subheadings to give a picture of the range of views that emerged (see Figure 11.3).

Although all quotes must be anonymized it may be necessary to identify individuals by their code number either to assure the reader of the dependability of your research or to show the development of views through the themes in different individuals. If you have interviewed different groups of people about the same issue you may

---

Theme 3: Perceived value of health care services
All the elderly people interviewed (23) found at least one aspect of the health care they received at the day hospital to be valuable.

3.1: Nursing care
Eleven people valued being able to have a bath at the day hospital. Six said they could not have managed in their own baths, even with help. Two people said they could only use the day hospital baths as the necessary equipment was not available to them at home. The majority of people who valued this service (10) appreciated having an experienced person on hand to assist them. Others simply expressed their pleasure at being able to make use of this facility.

'I look forward to coming here just to have a lovely bath.'

'The staff are very kind and efficient. I thought I would get embarrassed but they just make me feel so comfortable. It's a real pleasure.'

Figure 11.3   Example of how a section of the final report may appear using the content analysis example.

Theme 1: Accessing the day hospital
Interviewees had differing opinions about the ease with which the day hospital could be accessed.

'I had problems with my legs for months. I asked the doctor if I could come here to get it sorted out but he said there was a long waiting list and I would have to have the district nurse.' (Patient)

'We have good relationships with the local GPs with an open referral system for assessment.' (Nursing staff)

Figure 11.4   Example of identifying interviewees to show differing perspectives.

like to identify them by designation as you seek to explore views around the themes (see Figure 11.4).

Another way of showing different perspectives in a comparative format is to develop a matrix. The example in Figure 11.5 looks at the role of the community paediatric physiotherapy service from the perspective of parents of children with disabilities. This hypothetical example shows that parents of children receiving physiotherapy in a school with a special needs unit have different views to parents of disabled children in mainstream schools. For comparison a matrix is set up to reflect the views of each group. Each box summarizes the perspectives for each theme, then single quotes are entered here to illustrate the views. These would be expanded on in a final report.

Verifying the process and outcome of the analysis

Chapter 8 outlined the importance of the validity and reliability of the research process and Chapter 5 looked at how the interview process can be piloted to ensure this. It is equally important that the analysis of interview data undergoes rigorous scrutiny to ensure that the themes that are pulled out are trustworthy. Holloway and Wheeler (1996) argue that some researchers do not consider the terms validity and reliability to be appropriate in qualitative research. They prefer the terms credibility, transferability, dependability and confirmability, which they define as follows:

1. *Credibility:* ensuring that the participant group is accurately identified and described.
2. *Transferability:* enabling readers of the report to generalize the findings to other settings.
3. *Dependability:* checking that the research process is rigorously conducted.
4. *Confirmability:* judging whether the findings emerge directly from the data.

You can verify your analysis of interview data to take into account these four issues by rereading your scripts, verifying themes with colleagues, confirming themes from other data sources, leaving an audit trail or validating themes with participants.

Theme	Special unit parents' views	Mainstream schools parents' views
Availability and quality of physiotherapy	The same physiotherapist visits regularly three times a week. 'We are very happy. We know Jimmy is getting his physio even though he won't do his exercises at home.'	The physiotherapist visits by appointment once or twice a term. 'Obviously we would like more physio for Sarah but we want her to be at school with her local friends too.'
Availability and quality of school support staff	Two qualified children's nurses provide full-time nursing and therapy support. 'Mrs Williams puts her calipers on every morning when she gets to school then watches her walk to her classroom.'	Support varies between schools. Support staff are taught individual therapy programmes by the visiting physiotherapist. 'Lee gets a 20 minute session with the welfare lady when his class have games.'
Environment/ facilities	A dedicated special needs room is equipped with nursing, therapy and teaching aids. 'All the catheter stuff is there and the wheelchair man comes every term.'	Specialist equipment has to be purchased for each child. Funding is a permanent problem. 'We had to fund-raise to get a special chair for James.'
Parental involvement	There is no formal arrangement for the parents to meet with the physiotherapist. 'It happens on an ad hoc basis. I'd like something more formal.'	The physiotherapist always asks the parents if they would like to be present at each session. They usually attend. 'The physiotherapist lets me know when she is coming and we update his programme.'
Parental view of child's perspective	The children seem to like the routine and get to know the physiotherapist well. 'Tom loves her. He'll do anything for her.'	These children get much less formal therapy input but attend their own local school. 'We have to offset the amount of therapy against the advantages of attending a village school.'

Figure 11.5   Using a matrix to show different perspectives.

It is very easy to come to a research question with preconceived ideas about the answer. Not only is it possible to bias your interview questions but it is also possible to, deliberately or unwittingly, bias the analysis. To avoid potential researcher bias, read and reread your scripts to pull out all possible themes and perspectives (see Chapter 5).

Ask a colleague to read some or all of your scripts and identify themes. Discuss any differences in outcome and amend your categorization where appropriate. You could also leave an audit trail (Lincoln, 1985) by keeping a detailed project journal that allows others to check the rigour of your methodology and form a judgement as to the dependability of your findings.

Maykut and Morehouse (1994) recommend that you validate your themes against other possible sources such as observation and documentary evidence in order to 'lend strong credibility to the findings'.

Once you have transcribed and analysed an interview it may also be helpful to ask the interviewee to validate your interpretation. In the authors' experience most participants make only a few minor amendments. However, if your interviewee feels that you have made fundamental errors of fact and interpretation, it is necessary to revisit your field notes and transcription and decide whether your analysis is at fault or if the participant has changed his/her views since the interview took place. Discuss highly contentious or differing views with your supervisor or project manager before deciding whether to use them in your final report. It is not unknown for interviewees to make contentious comments at interview only to realize afterwards that these should have been 'off the record'. Although you assure interviewees of anonymity, they may worry that people reading between the lines of your report will be able to attribute quotes to them. It is important to respect these concerns.

Key points

1. Interview data may be analysed in many different ways. This chapter discusses three ways likely to be used by therapists in undergraduate or clinical research: content analysis, thematic analysis and grounded theory analysis.
2. Content analysis is a basic form of interview analysis often used in surveys and patient satisfaction projects. Results may take the form of consolidated answers to questions, illustrated by quotes.
3. Thematic analysis explores issues in more depth, allowing themes to emerge and testing their validity in subsequent interviews. Only themes of relevance to the research questions are put into the research report. These are illustrated with quotes.
4. Grounded theory analysis is a more rigorous process, allowing theories to develop based on the themes arising from the interviews. These theories are then tested in later interviews, allowing for modification or expansion. The report is based on the theories that emerge. Quotes may be used as evidence of confirmation of the theories.

5. Prior to analysis, data must be prepared. This includes transcription of tapes or typing of field notes and laying out the script to enable coding.
6. Scripts are coded by pulling out key words and drawing them into categories or themes. These may be refined or expanded as more scripts are analysed.
7. Analysing scripts immediately allows findings to inform subsequent interviews.
8. Verification of the process and outcome of the interviews involves assessment of credibility, transferability, dependability and confirmability.

References

Bowling, A. (1997). *Research Methods in Health: Investigating Health and Health Services*. Open University Press.

Clark, D. (1997). What is qualitative research and what can it contribute to palliative care? *Palliative Medicine*, **11**, 159–166.

Glaser, B. and Strauss, A. (1967). *The Discovery of Grounded Theory: Strategies for Qualitative Research*. Aldine.

Holloway, I. and Wheeler, S. (1996). *Qualitative Research for Nurses*. Blackwell Science.

Lincoln, Y.S. (1985). *Naturalistic Inquiry*. Sage Publications.

Maykut, P. and Morehouse, R. (1994). *Beginning Qualitative Research: A Philosophic and Practical Guide*. The Falmer Press.

Oliver, J. (1995). Counselling disabled people: a counsellor's perspective. *Disability and Society*, **10**, 261–279.

Payne, S. (1997). Selecting an approach and design in qualitative research. *Palliative Medicine*, **11**, 249–252.

Richards, L. and Richards, T. (1994). From filing cabinet to computer. In *Analysing Qualitative Data*. (A. Bryman and R.G. Burgess, eds), pp. 146–172. Routledge.

Seale, C. (1994). Qualitative methods in sociology and anthropology. In *Studying Health and Disease*. (K. McConway, ed.), pp. 22–35. Open University Press.

Segal, J. (undated). *Emotional Reactions to MS*. ARMS Education Service.

Strauss, A. and Corbin, J. (1990). *Basics of Qualitative Research: Grounded Theory Procedures and Techniques*. Sage Publications.

Complementary reading

Bryman, A. and Burgess, R.G. (1994). *Analysing Qualitative Data*. Routledge. Chapter 3: Analysing discourse.

Robson, C. (1993). *Real World Research: A Resource for Social Scientists and Practitioner-Researchers*. Blackwell. Chapter 12: The analysis of qualitative data.

Smith, J.A., Harré, R. and Van Langenhove, L. (1995). *Rethinking Methods in Psychology*. Sage Publications. Chapter 7: Basic principles of transcription.

Strauss, A. (1987). *Qualitative Analysis for Social Scientists*. Cambridge University Press.

Tesch, R. (1990). *Qualitative Research: Analysis Types and Software Tools*. The Falmer Press.

12　Analysis of observations

Different types of analysis

In Chapter 6 we covered issues surrounding the design of observations. Analysis of observational data is likely to be influenced by whether your observation is structured or unstructured. A very structured observation often lends itself well to a more statistical analysis whilst a more unstructured observation will suit a more exploratory approach to analysis. Therefore, before you start analysis you need to be very clear of your research purpose and your research question. This chapter will demonstrate some useful analysis techniques using two sample data sets. The first sample will be from an unstructured observational study and the second sample will be from a structured observational study.

Sample data from unstructured observational study

The purpose of this unstructured observational study was to investigate how microcomputers were currently being used with adults who have a severe learning disability (Seale, 1993). The study was exploratory in nature in that it wished to identify the key factors that influence successful microcomputer use. Pilot work involved the researcher visiting local departments and becoming a participant observer for one session a week over 10 weeks. Each observation session lasted three hours. For each session the observer would attend computer sessions, staff meetings and lunch hours. All the staff were aware that they were being observed. Data from two observation sessions will be presented in this chapter.

Exploratory analysis

An inspection of the raw data in Table 12.1 highlights a couple of useful points about the recording of observations. Firstly we can see that, as a participant observer, the researcher has been able to record information not only about what they have seen but also about what they have heard in direct and indirect conversations. Secondly, we can see that the information the researcher has recorded which is not directly relevant to computer usage may help us to place other observations into context. For example, in day two we can see that the researcher has recorded an observation of a lunch hour. The way staff interact with one another in their lunch hour may help us interpret or understand how they interact with one another in more formal situations. Finally, the raw data also show some evidence that the observer has made an initial attempt to do some cross-referencing of information. For example, in the second day of observation they record

Table 12.1   Indexed raw data from unstructured observation

DAY ONE: 21/4/88 Thursday afternoon

Conversation with manager: The centre has two computers. The first was bought in 1984/1983. This purchase was instigated by the Assistant Director of Nursing Services who visited SEMERC's (Special Educational Microelectronic Resource Centres) in order to draft a proposal for equipment. Advice was also sought from the local university and polytechnic. The second computer was bought by money raised by the Hospital League of Friends. The manager instigated the fund raising.   1, 2, 3

Observation: During computer sessions with clients the staff stay and work with the clients, usually having the individual program plan to hand. Daily records are kept of computer sessions under the headings of Activity, Objective, Equipment and Evaluation. There was a high staff-to-client ratio with four to five staff in the session. Four clients used the computer and when asked by me 'Do you like working on the computer?' they all said yes.   1, 5, 3

DAY TWO: 27/4/88 Wednesday afternoon

Overheard: The department is going to convert an alcove in one room into a computer room so that it is away from other activities and the clients are not distracted. (Where will the money come from?) The manager and one member of staff got the computer scientist to write software again this week. (Like last week the staff and manager are interacting with the expert.) What kind of software do they want? Adapting old software – want more stimuli, want to know whether the client is paying attention to the screen.   1, 3, 4

Observation: The computer scientist was running the computer sessions with clients, but not in isolation from the staff. The staff were overlooking what was going on in order to see how the clients were progressing. The computer scientist reported back to the staff on progress and the staff filled in the progress sheets. The session was set up especially to make use of the expert's time.   1, 3, 4

Conversation: Re League of Friends funding. The two departmental managers talked together about getting another computer; they then went to a League of Friends meeting to ask for the money. (All the staff attended this meeting – even one who was ill and had to come in specially – see day four). The League of Friends is now coming to look at the computer to see what they have bought. The manager is going to try and ask them for some more money for software. She feels they have enough software for their more profoundly handicapped clients and now need software for their 'Group Home' clients.   1, 2, 3

Observation: Lunch hour staff were very friendly and chatty, and even though they were on their break they were still talking about clients and asking advice. The staff were also helping trainees over lunch with their work. One staff member was reading an OU book on 'Self-educating'. The staff seemed happy to ask the manager about anything, e.g. holidays. The manager announced to all staff changes to one client's program even though they may not all work with this client. The manager was not aloof, had her lunch with staff.   4

Observation: Computer session with four clients, three members of staff, including the computer scientist. Up to five activities happen in the session, only one of which may be the computer. The computer session might only last five minutes. Time not recorded on the record sheet. Clients: partially sighted, wheelchair users. Staff ask the clients if they want a go on the computer and don't seem to force.   3, 5

Conversation: Problems in using computers include: Problems with record-keeping system – records of clients go all over the hospital, since many different staff work with the clients. Practically every piece of software needs adapting or changing. Not enough software for the blind. The manager considers the computer to be a complement not a substitute for a member of staff.   2 that a member of staff attended a meeting, despite the fact that they were ill. This seems to have some special significance and the observer has made a note to check the notes for day four of observation.

You will note that the data have been cross-sectionally indexed. That is, the same set of five categories (1–5) has been applied across the whole data set. For such a small data set it is probably not worth indexing the data, but for a large data set indexing may be useful to help you find instances of certain categories. While indexing may help you to organize your data, you will also need to make sense of what the codes 1–5 actually mean or correspond to. Table 12.2 outlines the five different coding categories with examples. The categories correspond to five factors that might influence computer use.

Table 12.2 From codes to categories

Category	Examples
Planning and decision making: Code 1	Assistant Director of Nursing Services drafted a proposal for equipment. Positioning of computer to reduce distractions. Special computer session to make use of expert's time. Two departmental heads discussing with each other whether to buy another computer. Recognition that need more software for group home clients.
Resources: Code 2	Second computer bought from League of Friends funds. Going to League of Friends to ask for money. Not enough software for the blind. High staff-to-client ratio.
Support: Code 3	Advice was sought from SEMERC, local university and polytechnic. Financial support from League of Friends. Getting computer scientist to write software. The session was set up especially to make use of the expert's time. Three members of staff, including computer scientist, involved in session.
Staff involvement: Code 4	Staff stay and work with clients, usually having individual program plan to hand. The manager announced to all staff changes in one client's program. The staff were overlooking what was going on in order to see how the clients were progressing. Staff and manager interacting with computer expert.
Computer use: Code 5	Daily records are kept of computer sessions. Time not recorded on the record sheet. Up to five activities happen in the session, only one of which might be the computer. The computer session might only last five minutes.

Table 12.3 From categories to subcategories

Factor category	Subcategories	Examples
Planning and decision making	Before obtained computer	Visiting SEMERC in order to draft proposal.
	After obtained computer	Plans to convert an alcove.
	Internal	Two departmental managers discussing purchase of another computer.
	External	Assistant Director of Nursing Services engaging in information gathering.
Resources	Staff	High staff-to-client ratio during computer sessions.
	Money	Funding from League of Friends.
	Hardware equipment	Two computers.
	Software equipment	Adequate software for more profoundly handicapped clients. Inadequate software for blind clients and clients in a 'group home'.
Support	Technical support	Help from a computer scientist in writing specialized software.
	Ideological support	Staff and management supportive of the idea that computer may be of benefit with client group.
	Internal support	Staff and management.
	External support	League of Friends. Computer scientist.
Involvement	Staff	Staff involved in working with clients on the computer. Staff involved with working with computer scientist.
	Management	Manager involved in computer use and interacting with computer scientist.
Computer use	Access organization	Four clients used the computer. Up to five activities happen in the session, only one of which might be the computer. The computer session might only last five minutes.
	Evaluation	Computer use recorded (time not recorded).

Now that we have identified five separate categories it may be possible to break these categories down a little further in order to identify themes or make more sense of why and how these factors are important. Table 12.3 outlines the breakdown of the five categories into subcategories. From that we can see some strong themes emerge. For example, 'internal' and 'external' emerge as subcategories for the categories of planning and support. 'Staff' emerges as a subcategory for both resources and involvement. These themes may help us to develop our ideas as to why these five factors influence computer use and to inform any follow-up work that is done following this pilot study. What the analysis has not attempted to do is to make links between the five identified categories. These links might merit further investigation. For example, the quality of the plans and decisions made regarding computer use may influence the amount of resources available to support computer use. Or the degree to which staff are involved in decisions regarding the computer may influence how supportive they are of computer sessions.

Sample data from structured observational study

The data in this example come from a structured observational study that was attempting to evaluate the learning outcomes of two computerized teaching programs (Galuschka, 1987). These programs were designed to be used with adults who had a severe learning disability. Experimental sessions involved comparing learning on two computerized tasks with learning on two similar non-computerized tasks. In order to conduct a comparison, participants were filmed whilst engaging in both the computerized and non-computerized tasks. These videos were analysed using a lap-top computer and a behavioural analysis program (Felce *et al.*, 1984). With this program the lap-top keys can be used to encode behaviours. In this study six behaviours were identified as being important and each was allocated a key (see Table 6.2 in Chapter 6). The observer would watch the videos and, when they saw a certain behaviour, they would press the appropriate key on the lap-top. At the end of the observation session the lap-top could produce a printout that gave analyses of sequences and duration of behaviours.

Before the whole set of videotapes could be analysed by two observers a small reliability study needed to be conducted in order to check whether the observers were applying the same category codes to the same behaviours. The observational records from one session were compared.

Descriptive and statistical analysis

Figure 12.1 shows what a computer printout from each observer's lap-top might look like. The shaded areas indicate occasions where observations from the two observers have exactly matched or overlapped. For example, observer 1 recorded inappropriate behaviour as occurring from the 64th second of the session to the 88th. Observer 2 recorded inappropriate behaviour occurring from the 65th second to the 87th second. In this situation there is an overall agreement of some 22 seconds.

An initial scrutiny of this raw data indicates several interesting points. Firstly you will note that the observer SB has observed reinforcement (Z) to have occurred whereas observer JK has not. This discrepancy means that SB has recorded more behaviours than JK (29 compared to 23). You will also note that on several occasions a behaviour is recorded as lasting for 0 seconds. There could be several reasons for this, including the fact that the behaviour lasted for milliseconds but the lap-top program could not record that, or the observer realized they had the wrong code and switched the key off fairly quickly.

Day: 1				Day: 1			
Client ID: MO				Client ID: MO			
Observer: JK				Observer: SB			
Ending time: 165				Ending time: 165			
Location: Hby				Location: Hby			
Session No: BL1.1S				Session No: BL1.1S			
Member of staff: DN				Member of staff: DN			
BEH	START	FINISH	DURATN	BEH	START	FINISH	DURATN
1*	6	7	1	1*	6	7	1
1	8	12	4	1	8	10	2
1	16	19	3	1	10	11	1
1	27	27	0	1	16	19	3
O	28	60	32	1	25	27	2
O	61	61	0	O	28	47	19
O	61	62	1	I	29	47	18
O	62	62	0	Z	30	31	1
O	63	63	0	Z	32	32	0
O	63	64	1	P	48	49	1
P	64	88	24	I	51	60	9
O	89	99	10	O	51	56	5
I	89	94	5	O	62	65	3
I	96	99	3	P	65	87	22
O	100	101	1	O	88	104	16
P	104	116	12	I	88	97	9
1	118	120	2	Z	91	92	1
I	126	133	7	I	98	100	2
1	130	134	4	P	104	119	15
O	134	156	22	P	125	135	10
I	135	153	18	1	128	129	1
O*	158	166	8	1	130	131	1
I	159	165	6	1	132	133	1
				O	134	157	23
				I	136	154	18
				Z	137	138	1
				O*	158	166	8
				I	159	164	5
				Z	162	163	1

Figure 12.1   Sample raw data comparing the recordings of two observers.

In a reliability study we wish to measure the amount of agreement between two observers. An initial examination of the number of agreements that occurred reveals that there were only two occasions where the two observers completely agreed (indicated by an asterisk in Figure 12.1). That is, they both identified the behaviour with the same code and recorded it as occurring for the same length of time. An investigation into the amount of agreement that occurred for each behaviour suggests a greater amount of agreement. Table 12.4 reveals that there was agreement for 92 of the 165 seconds.

It is possible to use a statistical test to calculate the proportion of agreement between two observers after chance agreement is removed from consideration. A common test that is used is the kappa reliability

Table 12.4   Total amount of agreement between two observers

Behaviour	Amount of agreement (seconds)
1 = Prompting	7
O = On-task behaviour	37
P = Inappropriate behaviour	34
I = Correct response	14
Total	92/166

Table 12.5   Sample agreement matrix for inappropriate behaviour

AA	AB	BA	BB	Total number of hours observed
22	1	1	48	
12	3	1	14	
	10	1	15	
			6	
			31	
34	14	3	114	165

AA = scores where both observers recorded the behaviour as occurring.
BB = scores where both observers recorded the behaviour as not occurring.
AB = scores where observer 1 recorded the behaviour as occurring but observer 2 did not.
BA = scores where observer 2 recorded the behaviour as occurring but observer 1 did not.

test (Cohen, 1969). A central part of that test is the drawing up of an agreement matrix. This matrix not only records when the observers agree that an observation did occur, it also records when the observers agree that an observation did not occur (see Table 12.5). The kappa reliability test uses these figures to calculate the observed proportion of agreements and compares this to the chance proportion of agreements. This calculation results in one number (test statistic). In this example the kappa statistic is 0.732. This means that 73% of judgements regarding inappropriate behaviour agreed (with chance excluded). This indicates a high level of agreement.

Key points

1. How you analyse your observations will depend on whether they were structured and unstructured.
2. An unstructured observation can be coded to reveal pertinent categories and subcategories.
3. A structured observation can be analysed using a computer in order to assess inter-rater reliability.

References

Cohen, J. (1960). A co-efficient of agreement for nominal scales. *Educational and Psychological Measurement*, **20**, 37–46.
Felce, D., DeKock, U., Harman, M. and Repp, A. (1984). *Using the Epson HX-20 as a fully self-contained unit for data capture and analysis*. Paper prepared for Conference on Microcomputers and Observational Data: Hardware, Software and Analysis, Thomas Coram Research Unit, University of London.

Galuschka, J. (1987). *A behavioural video analysis of computer assisted learning in adults with severe learning difficulties*. Third year project, Psychology Department, Plymouth Polytechnic.

Seale, J. (1993). *Microcomputers in adult special education: the management of innovation*. PhD Thesis (2 volumes), University of Keele.

13   Practical considerations

The academic and practical elements of research

As you will already have gathered from the preceding chapters, there are two key elements to undertaking any research project: the academic element and the practical element. The academic element involves the identification of the research question, the decision as to which methodology most appropriately addresses the question and issues around data analysis and statistical tests. It also involves deciding on the depth and generalizability of the research and where to disseminate the findings. The practical issues are much more fundamental and include such considerations as 'is my project feasible within the available time?' or 'is my project workable in this situation?'. The practicalities of the project may have an impact on the academic elements of the project such as choice of participating cohort or size of the geographical area to be investigated. This is particularly so in undergraduate projects where access to patients, clients, carers and therapists may be restricted. In projects for higher degrees or funded research other practical constraints may be those of time, available expertise and money. The academic and practical elements need to be considered in tandem as they are of equal importance in the research process. You may have a wonderful idea that translates into a great research question which promises to answer a major therapy question, but unless it is possible in practice your efforts will be in vain. This chapter considers some of the practical considerations behind the academic process.

Research preparation

Practical considerations when preparing to conduct a research project include brainstorming around a research question, identifying other stakeholders and reading around the subject. Each of these will be considered in turn.

Brainstorming around the research question

The academic process of devising a research question has been covered in Chapter 2. It is important to ensure that your research idea is driven by clinical practice or the professional literature rather than simply being based on the outcome of an 'intellectual exercise' (Partridge and Barnitt, 1986).

In practice you may only have the germ of a research idea, particularly if this research project is being undertaken as part of a degree course rather than in response to a burning desire to find the answer to a sticky clinical problem. You will need to turn that research idea or topic into a question that not only satisfies the academic requirements of your course but also the practicalities of obtaining the information, using it to answer your research question and producing the final dissertation. You may need some help with focusing ideas and topics into a research question. Your research supervisor or colleagues can help, or look again at Chapter 2. Do not attempt to start the project without having a question, for without a question you will never know when you have reached the answer and your project could go on forever!

People are usually very willing to talk with you informally about your research topic or idea. Approach clinicians, colleagues and self-help group committees to gain general background information and help you to more clearly define your research question – perhaps from different perspectives. Remember you cannot gather actual project data until you have ethical approval (where required). It is also important not to use up your potential research cohort by brainstorming your project with them all before you begin. If you are working in a clinical setting and are new to research it is advisable to make contact with someone who has previous research experience. Many NHS Trusts have a research and development unit or support group who can help. Alternatively, contact your local academic institution. If there is not a therapy school at your local university it may be appropriate to make contact with the medical school, school of nursing or department of social science depending on the type of research project you have in mind. The national therapy professional bodies have research and development departments and officers who can advise further.

Identifying other stakeholders

Projects undertaken as part of a degree fulfilment will need to follow guidelines or criteria set down by the awarding institution and supervising staff. Those who fund projects will have well-defined criteria for cost, time and sometimes research questions too. If you are employed as a research assistant, someone else may already have defined the research question or topic. In each of these scenarios other people will have a stake in the outcome of the research and will therefore want a say in how it proceeds. It is sensible to establish all the fulfilment criteria right at the beginning of the project. Make notes and ensure that the goal-posts do not keep moving.

Reading around the subject

Do not forget that your project will need to identify and investigate the background to the question with descriptions, comparisons and critiques of previous work in the field (see Chapter 2). The literature should also inform your methodology. In practice this means collecting and reading all your literature before you start data collecting. There is nothing worse than gathering all your data before you read the literature only to find that the methodology you have painstakingly used is universally condemned!

Large university libraries are geared up to the literature needs of researchers. This means that facilities to allow on-line and CD-ROM searches will be readily available. However, there may be pressures on the system and it may be necessary to book time on the data bases. Be prepared to pay for this in some places. Popular academic and professional journals are available in most university and postgraduate medical centre libraries and articles can be photocopied for research purposes. Others may need to be applied for through the inter-library loan system. Although this usually works very quickly, more obscure papers and departmental reports may take a lot longer. Do not underestimate this. One of the current authors once waited eight months for a research report to be found in New Zealand, by which time the project was all but finished! If you are in a hurry it is worth asking at your library if they know where the nearest copy is held. If it is in a specialist hospital library in the vicinity it may be quicker for you to make a visit than wait for the loan request to come through.

The professional bodies have library resources available to members. There are cost implications if you ask the information officer to conduct your search, although it may be possible to book a free slot if you are prepared to visit and undertake your own search (contact individual professional bodies for more information). You are recommended to undertake your own search locally first, contacting the professional bodies' information officers for more specialist information. You will need to provide a range of key words to assist in the search.

Other information for your project can be obtained using the Internet or seeking general information from relevant charitable or self-help groups. These can often be a valuable source of facts and figures about illnesses and the people who live with them, providing useful background information for your study.

Getting focused

Once you have clarified the research question it is important to be realistic about how much you can achieve with the time and resources at your disposal. It is very easy to get carried away with the project and get side-tracked; after all you will be meeting interesting people and reading new literature. Keeping a copy of your research question, project timetable and protocol pinned up in a prominent place is a useful reminder of the scope and time-scale of the project. When deciding the scope of your research it is important to consider various practicalities that will have an impact on your ability to undertake and complete the project.

The researcher

Whether you are the researcher or will be employing a research assistant you will need to consider issues of skills, time and interests. In considering the skills of the researcher you may need to ask:

1. What are the skills of the researcher?
2. Is this his or her first research project?
3. Is he/she familiar with the proposed methodology?

4. Is he/she experienced in the field under scrutiny or will he/she need time to get to grips with the therapy culture, management structure and jargon?
5. How much project management and researcher supervision will be necessary? Who will provide this? How will this work in practice?

In considering time issues you may need to address how much time is available to do the project. If the researcher is also working clinically or writing up their PhD (as often happens with research assistants) it may help to set aside dedicated time each week for the research project, otherwise 'fire-fighting management' sets in and it is easy for the research to fall behind schedule.

It is also important to ensure that there is no potential for a conflict of interests between the researcher and participants; for example, patients being treated by the researcher in his/her clinical job being entered into the research project.

The participants

A major issue in thinking about participants is how are you going to sample them. Blacktop (1996) relates sampling technique to Winnie the Pooh's propensity for eating all the 'hunny' in the jar to satisfy himself that the whole jar did indeed contain honey! Blacktop (1996, p. 6) states: 'There is no universal recipe for obtaining a good sample'. He identifies the main questions to consider when choosing a sampling process, namely:

1. What is being sampled?
2. What is the purpose of the survey or experiment?
3. What is known about the population?

The academic element of the research project will inform your sampling technique. For example, you may seek a random sample of patients or therapists to participate in your research to ensure a generalizable spread of results. Naturally, your sample will be limited by the parameters of your study. If you want to investigate field injuries in elite women hockey players, your sample will be limited to people who fulfil those criteria. Other projects will seek to gather a wide spread of views and need to stratify their sampling technique. For example, if you wanted to look at the impact of physiotherapy on incontinence problems in women who have attended for treatment over the last year, then you may deliberately split your cohort into age bands and ethnic groups, taking a random selection of participants from each.

Sometimes it is difficult to find a large group of people who fulfil your criteria although you know they exist somewhere out in the community. 'Snowballing' may be the answer here. For example, imagine your research question is 'What are the home care needs of people with multiple sclerosis (MS)?' It is unlikely that there will be a full register of people with multiple sclerosis in your local area and, although you could access people through the local MS Society branch or Social Services, this may exclude a whole group of people with MS who are not known to either. It may be possible, however, that some of these people with MS know others and can put you in touch. Although the advantage of snowballing is that you probably gain a broader sample, the disadvantage is that you cannot randomize. These issues need to be weighed up when deciding on your sample.

Practical elements may also inform your sample. Your inclusion and exclusion criteria may need to set geographical boundaries concomitant with those of the ethical committee approving your research. You may need to exclude participants for whom English is not a first language if you are conducting in-depth personal interviews and do not have the funding or facilities for translation. Appropriate and careful sampling is necessary to ensure generalizability of results and is important if you are using inferential statistics in your data analysis (Hicks, 1995). There are many different sampling techniques used in quantitative and qualitative research, and these are discussed in Bowling (1997) and Reed and Procter (1996), respectively.

In addition to considering how you will sample your population you need to ensure that you will have enough participants for your study. The academic considerations may state that you need x participants in order to achieve a statistically significant result and certainly you must aim for this if statistical significance is important to the study. Before you start your project, at the protocol stage, you will need to ascertain how many potential participants will be available and how many of these are likely to be amenable to participation. Consider other extraneous variables such as holidays which might reduce participation. Piloting your methodology will give you a good idea as to how easy or difficult it will be to recruit subjects. With the best will in the world clinicians often overestimate the number of patients that will be available to you. When you spend all day treating patients with strokes it is easy to think that you have dozens on the books. It is sensible to sit down with the clinician and go back through the appointment book to get a realistic view of numbers. Trawl back several months, even a year, to ensure you get a realistic idea.

Gaining access

Gaining access to potential participants may require you to get organized, negotiate permission, keep in touch, make accurate interpretations of promises of help and offer something in return.

Getting organized will involve making a list of all the places and things you will need access to for your research. These may include libraries, data bases, therapists, patients or other participants, medical or other records, equipment, venues for undertaking the research etc.

If you wish to gather data in managed areas such as therapy departments, residential care homes, special schools or even at self-help group meetings, it is vital that you negotiate careful access with the appropriate manager or gatekeeper. Gatekeepers are those key personnel who you are relying on to allow you access to resources and potential participants. Contact them to introduce yourself, describe your project and seek their assistance. Follow this up with a visit, which may involve giving a brief presentation to potential participants and a letter thanking them for their interest and support and outlining your proposed project intervention. Ensure that everyone who should know about your project actually does know about your project. Send information sheets to key individuals. For example, if you wish to involve people living in residential care it is necessary not only to seek access from the manager but also agreement from the residents' committee. Similarly, you will need permission from the head teacher of a special school and the consent of parents and children for a project involving such groups.

Most ethics committees will require written evidence of collaboration from key gatekeepers prior to giving ethical approval (see Chapter 14). The ethics committee will expect you to obtain consent from individual participants once the project is underway before you collect data from them. Do not assume that ethical approval gives you *carte blanche* to enter wards and start interviewing patients and staff. If you are invited into a department to collect data or use equipment make sure that you have permission from the senior staff member and agree an appropriate time that does not interfere with the bona fide activities of that department.

There is often a long time-gap between approaching gatekeepers and potential participants and actually gaining ethical approval. Keep your contacts informed or they may feel that you have lost interest in them and be reluctant to help you once you are able to start. Keeping in touch also allows you to act quickly if your expected cohort starts to dissolve. Projects have suffered severe delays when researchers failed to keep in touch with potential participants only to find that the original enthusiastic gatekeeper has moved on or a self-help group has folded, leaving the researcher stranded without a participant group.

Researchers will often instil great enthusiasm and receive wonderful offers of help. It is wise to check that these offers are not only genuine but also likely to materialize. Follow up any promises with full discussions and obtain a commitment in writing. With the best will in the world people will promise you assistance and support that, on reflection, they are unable to carry through. Check carefully that promises are based on full information. For example, projects have failed because the loan of specialist data-gathering equipment has been withdrawn when it became apparent that it was going to be used in patients' homes and not the therapy department as the manager initially thought. Good communications can prevent wires getting crossed and lead to a successful project.

People who have contributed to your research may be keen to know the outcome. It is only polite to repay helpful managers, gatekeepers or participants for their time and assistance (quid pro quo). Offer to send project reports or abstracts, give a presentation or write an article in a relevant journal or newsletter. Remember, you or another researcher may wish to approach them in the future and need to leave them with a positive impression.

Time-scale

Time has a strange way of disappearing during a research project. First you are thinking there is loads of time and the next thing you know your dissertation or report date is looming! Calculate a realistic time-scale and build in some leeway if you can. The following points need to be considered.

When planning your timetable do not underestimate the time required to gain ethics approval or funding. Many local research ethics committees meet once a month but some only meet quarterly. Some will allow amendments to be sanctioned by the Chair, whilst others will require you to wait for the next formal meeting to give approval (see Chapter 14). If you are seeking funding the time-lapse between being awarded the grant and the red tape wheels grinding into motion to allow you to access the money may be greater than you anticipated. Try to find someone who has been through the process in your area before and ask him or her for some inside information on potential delays.

If you have asked someone else to collect data for you, you may need to take their holidays or sick leave into account which will delay your data gathering. Decide whether you need to build time into your timetable for this, whether you can put the report date back or whether you need to seek another data gatherer. Be wary, people are often very enthused by your project and promise to gather data for you, but when it comes to the crunch they do not have the time to deliver!

Usually we use past experience to help us estimate data collection time. For example, you may wish to involve carers of people with new strokes in your project. Looking back through departmental records you see that typically you could expect three new patients a month. You therefore plan to interview the carers of ten new patients over the next three months, allowing for two drop-outs. However, when you come to the end of the data collection time you have only included four. This may be due to reduced numbers of patients coming through the unit, people having no immediate carer and people refusing or being unable to participate in your project. Running out of data collection time can be due to circumstances under your control, including poor estimation of participant availability, poor time management and poor project management. You may run out of time for reasons not under your control, such as unexpected low availability of participants, researcher sickness or other unexpected time out and deliberate lack of co-operation from people who initially gave willing consent.

Be realistic when estimating the time involved in data preparation, analysis and writing up. Take advice on this from your supervisor or other researchers. Take account of the availability of anyone else assisting in the data preparation and analysis, such as research assistants and statisticians or typists, in the preparation of your report. Never underestimate the time needed to transcribe interview data. An hour's interview can take an experienced transcriber one working day to transcribe! If you are sharing computers, book adequate time. Some establishments use networked computing systems which share software, especially expensive literature data bases, graphics and statistics packages. Allow time to get on to these. There is nothing worse than setting yourself a personally achievable deadline only to find you cannot access the necessary software. Remember systems can 'go down', especially when overloaded. It is not uncommon for printers to fail hours before dissertations are due for submission. Build in enough time to account for this or set up contingency plans for the 'worst case scenario'!

Check that participants are available at the time you require them. Think about holidays and busy times. Asking respiratory physiotherapists to attend a focus group during their busy winter workload will not elicit many participants. When calculating how much time it will take to administer a postal questionnaire do not forget to leave enough time for people to complete and return them. Build in enough time for follow-up questionnaires if there is a poor initial return. When planning interviews do not assume that the interviewees will all be available within the one short period of time you have set aside.

If you have a project supervisor who expects to read part or all of your dissertation, allow adequate time for them to do this, and for you to make any necessary changes.

Supervision

Never start a research project without some form or support system. This may be formal supervision from a supervisor or regular feedback sessions with a steering group. Developing informal but regular links with other researchers and managers can be a useful substitute in clinical research situations.

Supervisors

If you are undertaking a dissertation for a degree you will have a supervisor. It is usual to have one, maybe two, supervisors. You may have some choice or a supervisor may be allocated to you. In any case your supervisor should have some expertise in either the area you are researching or the methodology you will be using. If you are lucky they will have both. If your area of research is 'falls in the elderly', which you hope to investigate through a series of interviews, you can expect your supervisor to have care of the elderly or falls as an area of interest and expertise or be experienced in qualitative data gathering and analysis. Phillips and Pugh (1995) discuss supervision in depth with particular reference to undertaking a PhD.

Expect your supervisor to advise you on methodology, analysis and presentation. They may also read and comment on sections or all of your dissertation prior to final submission. Use them to brainstorm ideas and theories. They may also be able to put you in touch with other researchers in your field or smooth the way to gaining access to participants. In return they will expect you to turn up for appointments, take notice of what they say, not hassle them unduly and allow them to co-author any papers that emerge from your studies. The relationship should be one of mutual respect and not a long-distance acquaintance or a power struggle. It is worth sitting down at the beginning of the relationship to establish boundaries and expectations. Time spent doing this is rarely wasted. If you have two supervisors try to arrange dual supervision at least once or twice during your project. Clarify their roles and your expectations at the start of the project.

Other experts will doubtless be excited by your project and willing to advise on particular areas. For example, when investigating lower limb strength using isokinetic equipment you may have a supervisor who, although being knowledgeable in experimental research and good at the manipulation of numeric data, lacks expertise in the use of isokinetic rigs. Therefore you need to find someone to advise you on the equipment. Always keep your supervisor informed of the help you are getting from advisers and be careful that advisers do not slip into the role of supervisor, as this has great potential to muddle rather than illuminate!

Steering groups

Steering groups are commonly set up for funded research projects. The role of the steering group is to ensure that the research is kept on track, on time and within budget. There is no strict formula for the group's membership, although it is usual to include the key researchers, experts in different aspects of the research and perhaps a representative of the funding agency or participant group to be investigated.

An initial meeting at the beginning of the research is held to outline the project and discuss any pertinent practical and academic issues. The number of steering group meetings is decided at this meeting. Again, there is no strict formula, although it may be useful to meet at the end of each phase of data gathering and at the end of the project to discuss the final report before publication. It is usual in the latter meetings for the researchers to give a brief presentation/update on the research to the other members.

Steering group members can be used in a similar way to supervisors to gain advice on the academic elements and arrange introductions to potential participants. Group members may also provide useful contacts for future dissemination of results. Ensure that they get a free copy of the full, final report and a cup of tea at the meetings, there is rarely enough money in the budget to pay them for their time!

Project journals

Many researchers find it useful to keep a project diary or journal. In fact, your supervisor may recommend this approach. Project journals are best kept in loose-leaf folders so that you can easily make additions, although some people prefer to use a large, hard-bound notebook so nothing can get lost! The purpose of such a journal is two-fold. Firstly, it is a formal record of your project's progress and secondly, it is the recipient of all your wild thoughts, brainwaves and jottings.

A suggested journal structure is outlined below.

Formal section:
1. Project title and copy of the protocol.
2. Research questions/hypotheses (as appropriate).
3. Project plan.
4. Budget plan.
5. Time-scale and detailed timetable.
6. Actual day-to-day diary of research activities, appointments etc.
7. Supervisor's name and contact details or steering group details.
8. Adviser's name and contact details.

Informal section:
1. Names and numbers of useful contacts.
2. Brainwaves!
3. Lists of 'work to be done'.
4. Useful references and quotes.
5. Odd jottings (anything else that doesn't fit into any other category).

There will doubtless be times during your project when you become disillusioned and discouraged. Looking back at your journal and seeing just how much you have achieved can be very therapeutic. Having the research questions, timetable and budget so easily to hand helps to keep the project on track. Keeping all the information in one place in an easily identifiable format makes it easier to access than trawling through piles of paperwork on a shared desk! Make good use of this journal and you will reap the benefits when you come to write up your project as all your thoughts will already be captured and all you have to do is put them into the right order!

Never assume anything!

Research projects take organization and planning; you should never assume anything. Consider the following check-list to ensure that you have the necessary permissions and contacts to allow you:

1. Access to subjects.
2. Access to data/information.
3. Access to health measurement scales.
4. Access to facilities.
5. Access to assistant personnel, both research and administrative.
6. Access to equipment borrowed from companies or colleagues.

Turning a good research question into a good research project

The reality of doing research is that time spent planning is time well spent. Without good planning, what can go wrong probably will! Good project organization, timetabling and budgeting is vital. Make allowances for slippages and build 'catching up' time into your project plan. Accept that you may need to make changes to the protocol as you go along due to circumstances outside your control. These may include:

1. Altering the number of subjects.
2. Altering inclusion criteria.
3. Altering the methodology.
4. Altering the data collection procedure.

You will need to keep your supervisor or steering group, funders and the ethics committee informed about necessary changes. Ensure that you get your report in on time for marking or to the research funders or commissioners. If you need to seek an extension discuss this with your supervisor as early as possible as this may have implications for gaining your degree, or with funders as this may have an impact on your budget.

Poor planning can lead to:

1. Underanticipation of the size of the project.
2. Less than full appreciation of the realities of data collection.
3. Running out of time.
4. Running out of money.
5. Upsetting colleagues and participants.

Good planning can lead to:

1. Submission of a good project on time.
2. Continued support from colleagues, collaborators and participants.
3. A good reputation.
4. Future proposals being taken seriously.

Key points

1. Preparing for research includes brainstorming a research question, identifying the other stakeholders in the research, becoming familiar with the topic area, accessing the literature and addressing the practical implications.
2. Successful completion depends on being focused and organized. This includes accounting for the strengths and weaknesses of the researcher, the availability of and access to participants, and appropriate, feasible time-scales.
3. Research support may take the form of academic supervision, an expert adviser or steering group. Set parameters for this support early in the project to get the most out of it.
4. Project journals are a useful way of recording the progress of the project and noting ideas for future reference.
5. Never assume you have the necessary permissions to undertake the project. Ensure that you have promises of help in writing and keep participants and collaborators informed of your time-scale and progress.
6. Poor attention to practical detail can irritate collaborators and participants, leaving them reluctant to assist you or future researchers.
7. A good project is one that is well timed, well planned and well organized. Feed back your results to participants and collaborators as appropriate.

8. A good project increases the likelihood of your future proposals being taken seriously.

References

Blacktop, J. (1996). A discussion of different types of sampling technique. *Nurse Researcher*, **3**, 5–15.

Bowling, A. (1997). *Research Methods in Health: Investigating Health and Health Services*. Open University Press.

Hicks, C.M. (1995). *Research for Physiotherapists: Project Design and Analysis*. Churchill Livingstone.

Partridge, C. and Barnitt, R, (1986). *Research Guidelines: A Handbook for Therapists*. Heinemann.

Phillips, E.M. and Pugh, D.S. (1994). *How to Get a Ph.D. A Handbook for Students and Their Supervisors*. Open University Press.

Reed, J. and Procter, S. (1996). A sampling strategy for qualitative research. *Nurse Researcher*, **3**, 52–76.

Complementary reading

Drummond, A. (1996). *Research Methods for Therapists*. Chapman & Hall. Chapter 1: Preparation for research.

French, S. (1993). *Practical Research: A Guide for Therapists*. Butterworth-Heinemann. Chapter 6: Sampling and sampling designs.

14 Ethical and moral considerations

Defining research ethics

In a general sense ethics can be defined as the 'science of morality'. Those who are involved in this science are usually attempting to determine values for the regulation of human behaviour. From these values codes of ethics are applied and developed within particular professional contexts. For example, the field of medical ethics concerns itself with the relationship between the health care professional and patient. Issues such as giving bad news and abiding by patients' wishes are discussed within this field. When ethical codes are applied to professional contexts they are used to elaborate the perspectives and norms of the profession and are developed in order to maintain professional standards (Homan, 1991).

Widespread concern about the medical research undertaken by the Nazis during the Second World War led to the outlining of proper ethical principles involved in the acceptable use of human (and animal) subjects in research. In 1947 the World Medical Association established some guidelines for those involved in research involving human subjects. These guidelines were known as the 'Declaration of Geneva'. A formal code of ethics called the Declaration of Helsinki was published by the World Medical Association in 1964 and revised in 1975. This declaration was written specifically to cover medical research; however, many allied professional bodies have produced their own guidelines based on these declarations.

EXERCISE

Read the following four scenarios. For each scenario decide whether you think it raises an ethical concern and why. Try to rank the four scenarios in order, from the scenario that causes you the most concern to the scenario that causes you the least concern. What are the reasons behind your ranking? Compare your ranking with that of a colleague. Do you agree?

Scenario 1: A researcher spent two months observing five physiotherapists working in an outpatient department. He was looking at five different communication styles that the physiotherapists had. The researcher sat in with each physiotherapist on average twenty times during the two-month study. Five months after the observations had come to an end the physiotherapists contacted the researcher to enquire about the results of his study. The researcher reported that he was not going to publish the results because he had been unable to find any significant differences between the physiotherapists.

Scenario 2: A researcher advertised in the local paper for volunteers to take part in a study. He asked for people who had recently recovered from heart attacks to volunteer to come into his department and be interviewed about their experiences. Volunteers would be paid £20 for their time. Twenty people volunteered to come in. When they arrived in the department the volunteers were given their £20 immediately. When the interviews began, ten of the volunteers became unsettled at the nature of the questions and wanted to leave. The researcher tried desperately to get them to stay and even offered them more money to do so.

Scenario 3: A team of researchers were interested in trying out a new drug that they hoped would delay the onset of breast cancer in women who had been identified as having a high risk of developing the disease. The drug had never been used in humans but had been tested on laboratory rats. The team identified 100 women that they would like to include in their sample. These women were contacted by their GPs and asked if they would be interested in taking part in the trials. The women were told that the drug had not been tested on humans but that there were high hopes that it could be used to delay or prevent breast cancers.

Scenario 4: A researcher was interested in studying the leisure behaviours of adults who had severe learning difficulties. He arranged with a residential home to set up hidden cameras. The cameras were not placed in individuals' rooms but were placed in communal rooms, corridors and hallways. The researcher was interested to see how residents spent their leisure time and to look at the amount of time residents interacted with one another and with the home staff. The manager of the residential home gave permission for the cameras to be fitted, but the residents were unaware that they were being filmed.

Ethical issues concerning protecting the participant

Research often involves uncertainties, which may in turn involve risks for the participants. Such risks may include physical or psychological damage, loss of respect or dignity, infringement of privacy or exploitation.

A participant may be at risk from physical damage if the research is likely to injure them or illicit pain and discomfort. For example, asking a participant to take part in some step exercises for too long may cause an injury or cause the participant to feel some delayed pain the next day. Psychological damage may involve emotional upset, embarrassment or humiliation. Asking sensitive questions may cause upset or embarrassment. Sensitive questions might include those that ask about sexual behaviours or deal with a topic that the participant is not equipped to handle at that time. For example, if a carer is nursing a terminally ill relative it is probably highly insensitive to ask them questions about death and bereavement without good reason or proper negotiation.

The way a researcher treats research participants may influence whether or not they experience loss of self-respect or dignity. Asking a participant to complete a test or assessment where it is clear to everyone concerned that the participant either cannot complete the task or is getting everything wrong might well damage self-respect or dignity. None of us wants to be put in a position of feeling stupid in public. Treating the participant as inconsequential, a number on a list, rather than a person may also influence self-respect and dignity. People usually take part in research projects because they think they are doing some good. This may make them feel good about themselves and lead them to expect a researcher to be grateful or respectful. Of course we should all be grateful to participants who give up their valuable time to help us out, but often we don't show it.

A participant's privacy may be infringed in a number of ways. They may be asked to give information that is irrelevant to the study or of an overly personal nature. If a participant can be easily identified from information given in a public research report then privacy has not been respected. If information is collected in a covert way (disguised tests, hidden cameras, talking to third parties) then privacy is not being respected. Privacy may also be infringed if personal data supplied by participants is deliberately or accidentally 'shared' with others not involved in the research without the consent of the participant. As researchers we will all meet unusual or interesting characters that take part in our research. For example, you might visit someone in their own home in order to conduct an interview and discover that their home is, in your opinion, quite dirty and smelly. It might be pure purgatory for you to sit in their home for an hour wondering what kind of creatures are hopping on to your clothes and you may be dying to share that feeling of purgatory with your partner when you get back home. But, 'I met a man today who lived in a strange house' is less likely to be an infringement of privacy than 'I was at Mr Brown's house in Elton Road when I smelt this funny smell'!

A participant can be exploited in a number of ways. Researchers may put undue pressure on them to take part in the study. Or a researcher may take advantage of participants' willingness to help and recruit them to a study which in reality they cannot commit to. Participants may agree to take part in a ten-minute study only to find it actually lasts for an hour. The participant may belong to a 'vulnerable group' that can be easily exploited unless protected. This group may be vulnerable because it is over-researched or because the people who belong to the group are considered unable to give proper consent to take part in a research study. Such groups include children under eighteen, people with learning disabilities and those who are experiencing mental health problems.

The researcher must balance potential risks against potential benefits. He or she will be expected (by an ethics committee, for example) to demonstrate how participants will benefit from taking part in the research study, what controls will be taken to ensure the safety, welfare and rights of participants and how participants will be informed of potential risks. Three concepts that it is crucial to understand are informed consent, confidentiality and anonymity.

Informed consent

Sim (1986, p. 586) argues that prospective research participants must be given the 'fullest possible scope to protect his or her own interests'. The principle behind informed consent is that participants are given information about the study before the study takes place. Participants can then use this information to make an informed decision about whether or not they want to take part in the study.

Informed consent for research purposes is usually in a written format. Potential participants are given an information sheet that discloses information about the study. If the participants understand the information conveyed and are able to make a rational decision to volunteer to take part in the study, they then need to sign a consent form. The information sheet should include information about the researcher and the research and its implications for the prospective participant. Information about the researcher includes the name(s) and title(s) of the researcher(s) and the name and location of the institution where the research will be carried out. Information about the research includes the aims and purposes of the research (with a clearly stated title) and how the individual was selected to take part in the study. Implications for the prospective participant will include what the participant will be asked to do if they take part in the study, any possible risks in taking part in the study and what possible benefit taking part in the study will present to the participant. The information sheet should also include a statement that the participant is free to withdraw from the study at any time without giving a reason and without consequences, and an invitation to ask for more information (see Figure 14.1).

The consent form should have the title of the study clearly stated at the top. Such forms usually ask the participants to indicate whether they have read the patient information sheet, whether they have had an opportunity to ask questions and discuss the study, whether they have received satisfactory answers to all their questions and whether they have received enough information about the study. These questions are checking out whether the participant has been given enough information by the researcher. If the answer to any of these questions is no, then it is highly likely that the participant is not able to give informed consent.

Other questions on a consent form will check the participants understanding of what giving consent means and, where appropriate, what exactly the participant is giving consent to (being audio-taped for example). Examples of questions to include are: 'Do you understand that you are free to withdraw from the study at any time without giving a reason (or affecting your future medical care)?' and 'Do you agree to take part in the study?'. At the bottom of the consent form there should be space for the participant and the researcher to sign their names.

The presentation of written details should be supplemented by adequate oral discussion. Comprehension can be enhanced if the individual is allowed to take the information sheet and consent form

---

Occupational therapists' perception of clinical reasoning and its manifestations within care of the elderly

My name is Sally March; I am a second year occupational therapy student at the University of Southshore. I am in the process of carrying out a research study into clinical reasoning. The aim of the study is to identify the nature of clinical reasoning in the elderly care setting and to explore therapists' awareness and understanding of clinical reasoning. In order to find this out I hope to interview a small number of occupational therapists practising in the elderly care setting:

1. The interview will only take 45 minutes to an hour and will be conducted in a place chosen by participating therapists.
2. The interview will be tape-recorded (with permission from each therapist). The interviews will take place during July/August 1998.
3. Therapists' names, hospital names and any patient names will not be identified in the study report.
4. Transcripts of the interview will be forwarded to participating therapists for validation.

Participants will be free to withdraw from the study at any time and do not need to answer all the questions asked. As this is a student project, the results of this study are unlikely to change or influence occupational therapy practice generally. However, participating therapists may have a personal interest in the results and a summary will be available for inspection on completion of the study.

Figure 14.1 Example of an information sheet.

away before signing. Despite signing a consent form individuals have the right to ask questions and withdraw at any time. If the participant is unable to give informed consent (e.g. a child or someone with a learning disability) then it may be obtained from a relative or guardian (see Figure 14.2).

In addition to obtaining consent a researcher will often need to seek permission from various parties. If your study involves hospital patients, then permission will need to be sought from the patients' consultant. If your study involves healthy volunteers, a letter to their general practitioner can often help you identify if there is any reason why the person should not take part in your study. If you wish to use medical records, then permission must be obtained from the professional who is responsible for the care of the person involved. The researcher must provide details of the individuals who will gain access to the information and the procedures in place to ensure that there will be no disclosure to anyone else. Permission from line managers may be necessary for such things as interviewing people in work time, asking people to distribute questionnaires on your behalf and recruiting staff help with identifying and approaching potential participants on your behalf.

Sometimes it is not necessary to gain informed consent. For example, you do not need to get questionnaire respondents to sign a consent form. In this case, it is considered that respondents demonstrate their consent by completing the questionnaire. If they do

---

Occupational therapists' perception of clinical reasoning and its manifestations within care of the elderly

1. Have you read the information sheet?	YES/NO
2. Have you had an opportunity to ask questions about the study?	YES/NO
3. Do you understand the purpose of the study?	YES/NO
4. Do you understand that this is a student project that will result in a dissertation that will be marked?	YES/NO
5. Do you understand that you are free to withdraw from the study at any time and without giving a reason?	YES/NO
6. Do you agree to take part in the study?	YES/NO
7. Do you agree to your interview being audio-taped?	YES/NO

Signed..   Date..............................

Name in block letters...

Signed (researcher)....................................   Date..............................

Figure 14.2   Example of a consent form.

not wish to consent then they can simply not complete it or throw it in the bin. In other cases, researchers need to deceive participants about some aspects of the research for fear that knowledge would influence behaviour and hence results. Informed consent in these circumstances is problematic. For example, if you wish to observe a class full of students you are more likely to see natural behaviour if they are unaware that they are being observed. This kind of deception raises ethical concerns about using people. These concerns can be reduced by such measures as debriefing participants at the end of the study. Whilst debriefing might be seen as honest and ethical, there is no guarantee that the participants will not be upset. Someone may feel that by being deceived they have been made to look stupid or foolish.

Anonymity and confidentiality

Sometimes it is not necessary to ask a participant to divulge their name or to identify which participant gave which response. In these cases anonymity is offered by a study. In other studies a researcher is able to identify participants names and match names to responses. In these cases the researcher needs to assure the participant that this information will not be publicly divulged. Such assurances are assurances of confidentiality. Safeguards to confidentiality include coding identifying information, keeping identifying information in a secure place (locked cabinet or case) and destroying identifying information such as audio tapes at the end of the study. Giving assurances of anonymity and confidentiality can secure co-operation from potential participants and offers the researcher some protection from criticism or complaint.

Ethical issues concerning professional behaviour

A large part of convincing a potential participant or an ethical committee that you are capable of acting in an ethical manner involves convincing them that you can act in a professional manner. If you appear to be unprofessional then why should anyone trust you to be ethical? What constitutes professional behaviour in terms of research ethics is quite varied, but the following advice should stand you in good stead.

Make sure your letters contain no typing or grammatical errors. Such mistakes imply sloppiness and lack of attention to detail. Try not to be overly familiar or appear condescending. Make sure questionnaires and letters have a heading with the title of your project. Provide a contact address or telephone number where people can approach you if necessary.

Avoid making assumptions about permission or consent. For example, if a superintendent physiotherapist gives you permission to interview his or her staff, this does not mean that the staff have to agree to be interviewed. Getting ethical approval from an ethics committee does not give you any right to demand access to data or institutions or bypass the normal courtesies. If you appear arrogant in that you expect people to help you or are ungrateful for the help you receive, then it may have implications for the amount or nature of data that you obtain. People may also complain that you are acting 'unethically'. Such complaints, if carried through, may mean that you cannot finish the study, are unable to publish the results or that future funding may be put in jeopardy.

Acting in a professional manner may involve creating a positive, collaborative atmosphere in which participants and collaborators feel that they have a stake in the study and are not being used to promote your own individual glory. This might be achieved by involving collaborators in the design of your study or asking their opinions as to what they think will or will not work. Collaborators may wish you to include measurements in your study that will provide results that are of particular interest to them. It is well worth negotiating. If a head OT is going to hand out questionnaires on your behalf, which evaluate her service, why shouldn't she ask for certain questions of her own to be included?

French (1993) argues strongly that a large part of acting in a professional manner concerns what you do with the data once they have been collected. French argues that it is unethical to involve participants in a study and then not publish the results. In a sense, you will have wasted the participants time (used them) for no apparent purpose or benefit. It can be tempting not to publish results when they are statistically insignificant, unexpected or do not support your hypothesis. However, only publishing statistically significant results can bias and distort knowledge. Sometimes once a study is complete we can reflect on our design and methodology and realize the flaws and mistakes we have made. Seeing such flaws may make us reluctant to publish. However, we have a professional and ethical duty to help others learn from our mistakes. Make the shortcomings in the study known and identify how your study can be improved. In that way, the participants' valuable time will not have been wasted.

Other issues involved in dealing with data include falsifying or omitting results and making fraudulent claims about what your data prove or disprove. For some researchers it can feel as if they have staked their whole reputation on getting a certain predicted result. When that result cannot be obtained it can be very tempting to 'cook the books'. Altering data may solve the initial problem of protecting your reputation but it will be damaged sooner or later when other researchers fail to replicate your results and start to question your methodology and findings. Conducting research so often becomes a personal crusade and we can forget the source of the information that we are 'playing god with'. Research data evolve from participants who have worked with you (not for you) in good faith.

Method-specific ethical issues in research

In the previous section we discussed general ethical issues. There are also ethical issues that are specific to individual quantitative and qualitative research methodologies. For example, in quantitative research, randomized controlled trials (RCTs) are often discussed in terms of the ethical dilemmas they pose. Sim (1989) identified three major ethical dilemmas with RCTs. Firstly, there is a dilemma surrounding withholding a new therapy from the control group, with possible loss of therapeutic benefit. Secondly, there is the problem of withholding a standard therapy from the experimental group, again with possible loss of therapeutic benefit. Finally, there is the risk that the new, unproven intervention that the experimental group experience may have unknown side-effects. Sim offers a solution to this dilemma. He argues that a controlled trial should only be used if the relative efficacy of the novel therapy and standard therapy are genuinely unknown. If the benefits of a treatment are unknown then it must be demonstrated that the risk to the participant is negligible. Placebos are often used with control groups in RCTs. A placebo is an inert form of treatment that is administered in order to equalize the 'psycho-physiological' effect of being treated between the groups. It can be argued that employing placebos without informed consent has serious ethical implications. Sim (1989) suggests that a case may be made for the use of a placebo when there is no recognized effective standard therapy.

If a participant is randomly assigned to a group then it may be argued that their autonomy has been overlooked in the interests of experimental expedience. A hidden assumption with randomization is that participants have no interest in which group they are assigned to. Sim (1989) highlights the argument that if randomization is a key element of a RCT it should form a key part of the information given to a participant. In clinical research, many feel that the requirements of random allocation can distort the therapist–patient relationship.

Ramos (1989) discussed the ethical implications of qualitative research. She argues that the characteristics of qualitative investigation seem to generate particular decision-making problems for the investigator who seeks to safeguard the research participant. Such problems include subjectivity, informed consent and confidentiality. A key element in most qualitative research is the relationship between the researcher and participants. Within this relationship boundaries can become less clear and so, for example, the role of the researcher may be confused with that of friend, therapist or adviser.

The discussions of the ethical issues within ethnography (Lipson, 1994; Baillie, 1995) also focus on the relationship between researcher and participant. They warn of the dangers of exploiting relationships for a purpose that cannot be fully understood by the informants. One commonly recognized problem is that of informed consent. Language and cultural factors are frequent barriers to an informant's real understanding of what it means to participate in a study and who can consent for whom. Because ethnographic studies evolve over time, a researcher cannot predict what questions they may ask or what risks may be involved in the future. There is perhaps a need for what is called 'process consent' whereby consent is reviewed and changed several times during a study.

Smith (1995) focused on the ethical issues surrounding the use of focus groups. One issue is that of over-disclosure by group participants. Within focus groups, participants reveal themselves to each other as well as to the researcher. Here, not only does the researcher need to respect privacy and confidentiality, but so too do the group members. Focus group researchers cannot promise or ensure strict and absolute confidentiality because they do not have control over what participants may disclose after they leave the group. But the researcher can inform participants that this may occur and can include in an information sheet comments that acknowledge this potential problem. The intensity of the interaction of the group may be stressful to some members of the group or they may find the topic of the focus group too sensitive. Researchers therefore need to be aware of how participants may be feeling when they leave the group. One solution is to provide a debriefing component to the session so participants can discuss their reactions. Or the researcher could allow a few minutes for the group members to debrief informally after the session. During the focus group the researcher may need to monitor the stress levels of the group and intervene accordingly.

Ethical committees

Most research that involves patients or health care staff is likely to be submitted to an ethical committee attached to a health authority for approval. Each committee will cover a specific geographical area and will consider itself responsible for protecting all people within that area, irrespective of whether they are hospital patients or not. Some organizations such as Social Services have their own regulatory bodies. Students may need to submit an ethical proposal to a university or college ethics committee. Medical ethics committees are usually multi-disciplinary and consist of doctors, nurses and lay people. Unfortunately, inclusion of therapists in such committees varies.

All cases of medical research involving human subjects, including the use of foetal material, embryos and tissues from the recently dead, should come before a full ethics committee. There may be some research that does not pose any evident ethical problems and therefore does not require submission to an ethical committee. For example, research where there is no risk of distress or injury to the subjects such as questionnaire surveys. French (1993) argues that, while some studies may not need approval by a committee, it is the responsibility of the researcher to find out what is required. Sometimes, however, it is not always clear whether your study needs ethical approval. In these circumstances perhaps it is better to be safe than sorry. Submitting to an ethical committee may help to highlight ethical issues that the researcher has not seen. Researchers can become so immersed in the objectives and purpose of their study that they can lose sight of the impact and practicalities of the study. Your local ethics committee can give you advice about using vulnerable groups and often have a register of groups that are 'over-researched' within the area. Furthermore, they may be able to put you in contact with useful people such as interpreters. Finally, the acceptance of research papers by many journals is often conditional upon submission to an ethical committee.

Ethical committees have no direct sanctions. But if an investigator bypasses or ignores the recommendations of an authorized ethical committee they may be vulnerable to professional disciplinary or legal proceedings.

The function of an ethics committee

There are often misconceptions surrounding the function and scope of an ethics committee. Bage (1992) discusses the scope of a medical ethics committee. Firstly, it has to advise its appointing authority on all matters pertaining to the ethics of research involving human subjects. Secondly, it must review all proposals for research to be carried out in the institution or area of authority. It may also review proposals for research to be carried out by staff of the authority in other places where there is no ethics committee. Finally, it may make reports to the appointing authority, which are usually available to the public. These tasks help ethical committees achieve such objectives as maintaining ethical standards of practice in research, protecting subjects of research from harm, preserving subjects' rights, providing reassurance to the public and protecting researchers from unjustified criticism.

The criteria that ethical committees use for considering ethical proposals are often misunderstood or shrouded in mystery. Some of the main criteria of ethical committees are informed consent, confidentiality, selection and recruitment of subjects and evidence of permission from all relevant parties. Horner (1993) discusses the criteria for decision-making in local research ethics committees

(LRECs) in the United Kingdom. He discusses the criteria of identifying bad research. Bad research is considered to be unethical. What can be controversial, however, is what some people and committees consider bad research to be. As a general rule, bad research has a question that is not worth answering, a methodology that will not answer the question being asked and is considered not to be 'good science'.

The process of submitting to an ethical committee

Ethical committees meet at set times during the year, usually monthly. Each committee will have a standard ethics form that they expect applicants to complete. This form will need to reach the committee secretary or chairperson at a set time before the meeting. An ethical committee may expect multiple copies of the form to allow all members of the committee to have a copy of your proposal. The committee will meet to discuss the proposal and come up with a decision. Sometimes you may be invited to attend a 'viva' to answer questions about your proposal. There are also some occasions where the chair of the committee might feel able to give what is called 'chair's action'. This is where the chair is willing to approve your submission without it being presented to the full committee. Circumstances where this might happen are when other committees have considered your proposal or where the research is considered not to pose a major risk to participants. The decision from the committee might be approved, approved subject to amendments or withheld. You will usually be informed of the decision by letter. The amount and quality of the feedback given by ethical committees varies however.

Broader issues in regulating research

The process of trying to gain ethical approval for a project can highlight broader issues of concern or debate. These issues may not be strictly ethical issues and may be argued to be political in nature; nevertheless it is important to acknowledge that they exist. We will focus on the six main issues of professional self-interest, right and wrong, ultimate responsibility, student projects, racism and sexism and sponsorship.

Issues of professional self-interest

Whilst ethical codes are set up to protect the rights of individuals there is often an element of self-interest on the part of the researcher. Ensuring that your research is ethical takes up so much energy that, it is argued by some, researchers only make the effort because they have something to gain. For example, Homan (1991) argues that some researchers may play the ethical game not because they are concerned about the participants but because ethical treatment yields better results than unethical treatment. Research participants will be less co-operative if they feel they are being tricked or used. In an ideal world we should embark on the process of gaining ethical approval because we firmly believe in all the principles that the ethical committee is trying to uphold.

Issues of right and wrong

No matter how stringent the guidelines or the process of submitting and approving an ethical proposal, there is no absolute right and wrong. Some degree of subjectivity cannot fail to infiltrate the ethical process. For example, it is not unheard of for a researcher to submit the same ethical proposal to different ethical committees, be accepted by one of them and rejected by another (Bower, 1994). Which committee was right? They clearly were operating under different values. For example, some committees will not accept qualitative studies while others will. In these circumstances submitting ethical proposals becomes more of a political exercise than an ethical one.

Issues of ultimate responsibility

Critics of ethics committees argue that ethical committees absolve researchers from making ethical decisions. Homan (1991) argues that, because ethical values are not black and white and do change over time, the ultimate responsibility for ethically acceptable research must lie with the researcher. If this is true then the researcher carries a heavy responsibility that will test their integrity and professionalism to the limit.

Issues surrounding student projects

There is growing alarm amongst ethical committees at the number of undergraduate projects being undertaken. This is because there is concern that research participants may be over-researched or that more important funded research will suffer from a lack of volunteers. Ethical committees often argue that student projects have a dubious validity because they are of no immediate benefit to participants and are often only confirming known findings. Therefore, there is a danger that therapy schools will be pressurized into changing their research training so that students never get an opportunity to learn from real experience.

Issues of racism and sexism

In race and ethnicity research, questions of ethics and values are especially prone to controversy. For example, Stanfield and Rutledge (1993, p. 27) argue that predominantly white male researchers are interpreting racial issues in the USA. This is considered to have led to a number of 'disturbing value biases in race and ethnicity studies'. Horner (1993) notes that many ethical research committees do not adequately reflect ethnic minorities in their representation. He argues that it is unacceptable for a committee composed entirely of the host community to approve a research protocol that is to study the migrant community. The committee membership must be augmented, or the views of ethnic elders sought.

Eichler (1988) identified four main sexist problems in research: androcentricity, overgeneralization or overspecificity, gender insensitivity and double standards. She argues that these problems can occur at any stage in the process from posing the question to interpreting the results. These problems may raise ethical or political concerns. For example, ignoring sex as a socially important variable (gender insensitivity) or measuring identical behaviours in men and women by different means (double standards).

Gender issues do not simply involve sexism but also sexuality. For example, Warren (1994) discusses gender issues in field research. If a researcher becomes an integral part of a community then it is likely that they will come across issues of sexuality. These issues may involve others but equally could involve themselves. Warren is worried about what he calls a modern 'confessional impulse' to report sexual encounters that are not 'analytically salient'. Such confessionals may cross ethical, political and professional boundaries.

Sponsorship

Being sponsored by an organization to conduct research may produce some ethical dilemmas for researchers. Researchers may be expected to find and publish only those results that suit the organization's purpose. For example, a drug company may not be too pleased to hear that its drug does not perform well compared with other drugs. Sponsorship deals may require the researcher to sign a contract which gives the sponsor sole control over whether and how the results are disseminated. Some researchers may face a dilemma in that they need a company's money in order to carry on their research but do not actually approve of what the company does (e.g. a tobacco or drugs company).

Key points

1. The potential risks for participants taking part in research include: physical or psychological damage, loss of respect or dignity, infringement of privacy or exploitation.
2. Informed consent, anonymity and confidentiality can protect the participant.
3. Potential ethical issues concerning professional behaviour include: sloppy presentation, making assumptions about consent, collaborating with participants, publishing results and fiddling the data.
4. Individual qualitative and quantitative methodologies have associated ethical concerns; for example, randomized controlled trials, ethnography and focus groups.
5. The functions of an ethical committee are to maintain ethical standards and protect subjects and researchers.
6. Issues which broaden our thinking about ethical research include: professional self-interest, right and wrong, ultimate responsibility, student projects, racism and sexism and sponsorship.

References

Bage, B. (1992). Ethics committees and their role in clinical research. *Health Law Bulletin*, **16**, 3–4.

Baillie, L. (1995). Ethnography and nursing research: a critical appraisal. *Nurse Researcher*, **3**, 5–21.

Bower, E. (1994). Editorial: Ethicology. *Child Care, Health and Development*, **20**, 215–217.

Eichler, M. (1988). *Non-Sexist Research Methods: A Practical Guide*. Allen and Unwin.

French, S. (1993). *Practical Research: A Guide for Therapists*. Butterworth-Heinemann.

Homan, R. (1991). *The Ethics of Social Research*. Longman Inc.

Horner, J.S. (1993). Criteria for decision-making in local research (ethics) committees. *Public Health*, **107**, 403–411.

Lipson, J.G. (1994). Ethical issues in ethnography. In *Critical Issues in Qualitative Research Methods*. (J.M. Morse, ed.), pp. 333–355. Sage Publications.

Ramos, M.C. (1989). Some ethical implications of qualitative research. *Research in Nursing and Health*, **12**, 57–63.

Sim, J. (1986). Informed consent: ethical implications for physiotherapy. *Physiotherapy*, **72**, 584–587.

Sim, J. (1989). Methodology and morality in physiotherapy research. *Physiotherapy*, **75**, 237–243.

Smith, M.W. (1995). Ethics in focus groups: a few concerns. *Qualitative Health Research*, **5**, 478–486.

Stanfield, J.H. and Rutledge, M.D. (1993). *Race and Ethnicity in Research Methods*. Sage Publications.

Warren, C.A.B. (1988). *Gender Issues in Field Research*. Sage Publications.

Complementary reading

Currier, D.P. (1990). *Elements of Research in Physical Therapy*. Williams and Wilkins. Chapter 4: The proposal and ethics.

Drummond, A. (1996). *Research Methods for Therapists*. Chapman & Hall. Chapter 1, Section 3: Ethical considerations.

15 Writing a research proposal

What is a research proposal?

For any research you do, no matter how big or small, simple or complex, it is wise to prepare a statement about what you intend to do and how. This statement is known as a research proposal or protocol. Currier (1990) defines a research proposal as an organized plan of the proposed research. In comparing a researcher to an architect, Robson (1993) highlights the value of research proposals. A researcher draws up plans to investigate issues and solve problems. In each case these plans may say something about structure, about how the task is conceptualized, and about the methods to be used in carrying out the plans.

Why might you need to write a research proposal?

You may need to write a research proposal when you are thinking about conducting some research of your own. You may be a student conducting an undergraduate or postgraduate project. You may be a clinician conducting research as part of your work. Whatever the reason, putting your research plan on paper enables you to see if you have an answerable question and a viable method. It is advisable to write a research proposal regardless of whether or not you are attempting to gain funding for project. Indeed, writing a proposal may help you decide if you need funding. You can also show written plans or proposals to other people to get their comments and advice. Writing a proposal also helps you identify an appropriate time-scale or timetable.

Writing a proposal may help the researcher by identifying the research question and purpose of the proposed project, providing a guide for the researcher to follow while conducting the project and establishing limits and criteria to be followed and adhered to throughout the project.

Writing a proposal that can be reviewed and judged by others may also be useful in terms of providing a measure of accountability, having something to show to potential research participants, ethics committees and funding bodies and reducing error and preventing important aspects of the study from being overlooked.

Who may read your research proposal?

Robson (1993) argues that because research is an activity that is essentially in the public domain, it is appropriate that any proposed research should be open to inspection, comment and approval by others. Who those others may be will probably depend on why you have written the research proposal. They are likely to include such people as lecturers who are marking and supervising student research projects. A steering group or committee may review projects being undertaken as part of a clinical programme. Funding agencies will send proposals to internal reviewers or other external agencies. Prospective participant populations or guardians of the participant populations such as consultants, general practitioners, ward sisters, superintendent physiotherapists or head occupational therapists may wish to see a research proposal in order to decide whether to give permission for the project to go ahead. Ethical committees often like to see the research proposal in addition to their standard ethical form.

Whoever reads your proposal is likely to use a range of criteria to judge your proposal. A primary concern for many reviewers is whether the project has what is often called 'scientific value'. This refers to the merit or importance of the proposed project. What has merit or importance will depend on many factors such as the current research agenda of the day and accepted and proven research methodologies. Your proposal may also be judged on its value or contribution to a body of knowledge, the competency of the investigators, the appropriateness of the chosen methodology, the availability of facilities and resources (time, space, funds, equipment, personnel) for conducting the project and adherence to ethical and moral principles.

What is involved in writing a research proposal?

Our first instinct when answering this question is to say a lot of hard work! This is not meant to put you off, but simply to warn you that a good proposal takes some time to put together. This is because there is a lot of background work involved before you get to the point of writing your ideas down on paper or in a form. Depending on the nature of your research project you will need to conduct a literature search in order to find out what has been done before, to identify gaps in knowledge and to provide a theoretical and methodological background to the project. You will need to arrange meetings with all prospective parties such as potential collaborators, supervisors and participants (or guardians of participants), as well as institutional administrators or managers. You will need to discuss with these people issues such as design, costings, permission and division of responsibilities and tasks, along with the feasibility and practicalities of the project. Don't underestimate the importance of such meetings, they could make or break your project. Now is the time to involve colleagues or others who are going to play a part in your project, by collecting data for example, or administering the intervention. Finally, you will probably be required to complete a research proposal form. The proposal form you complete will look different depending on whether you are attempting to gain funding from an official agency, pass a student assignment or conduct a small study at work.

Table 15.1   Common elements of a research proposal and associated questions

Proposal section	Associated questions
Title	WHAT do you want to study?
Name of investigators	WHO is going to conduct the study?
Summary	WHAT do you want to study and WHY is it important that you study it?
Literature review	WHAT is the relevance of the study and WHAT is the current knowledge base in this area?
Problem statement	WHY is the study needed?
Research question	WHAT do you want to study?
Population	WHAT population will you be using to draw your participants from?
Definition	WHAT are your terms of reference?
Assumptions/limitations	WHAT factors will influence the outcome of your study?
Design	HOW are you going to try and answer your research question?
Equipment/instrumentation	HOW are you going to collect the data?
Selection of participants	WHO will be your participants and HOW will you recruit them?
Collection of data	HOW will you collect data, WHEN will you collect data and WHERE will the data collection take place?
Analysis of data	HOW will you analyse the data and attempt to answer your research question?
Time-scale	WHEN will each stage of the research project take place?
Costings	HOW much will the study cost?
References	WHY is the project relevant and worthwhile doing?

Completing a research proposal form

Whatever form you complete it will be attempting to get you to address several questions. What do you want to research? Why do you want to conduct the research? How are you going to conduct the research? When are you going to conduct the research? Who is going to be involved in the research?

The common elements of most research proposal forms are identified in Table 15.1, along with the associated questions that need to be addressed for each section. When you write a research proposal it will help if you always keep in your mind the who, what, when, where, why questions highlighted in the table. The following pages take you through, in more detail, what information may be required in each of the sections.

Project title

Give a descriptive title that easily identifies the project. In most cases it is not expected that this will be the final, definitive title of your dissertation or research report. The words in the title should be concise yet sufficient to give the reviewer a good idea of what the project is about or what is being proposed for study. The title may reflect the nature of the primary problem being addressed by the project.

Name and title of investigators

List all the investigators in order of contribution to the study and give an indication of their scholarly ability or competence. You may be required to name the research participants at the beginning of the proposal, together with their qualifications, work and research experience and particular expertise for the job. Funding agencies are often interested in where the investigators work in order to assess the reputation of the host institution and therefore the likelihood of the research being completed successfully.

> **Example of information given about investigators**: The research team is multi-disciplinary in nature, has a proven research background and experience of working with the target population. The team is ideally placed with members representing DoWell University and DoWell Community Health Trust. Jan Sealion PhD is a psychologist and has five years' experience of using the proposed methodology. Christine Oasis MA is an occupational therapist who has experience of working with the proposed client group. Caroline Royce PhD is a physiotherapist who works as a Research and Development Officer for DoWell Community Health Services.

Project summary

Indicate the likely importance and relevance of your project to health care and therapy. This is particularly important if applying for funding, where the aims and objectives of your project need to address the philosophy of the funding body. For example, in the UK if you are seeking funds from a regional department of the National Health Service Executive (NHSE) you will need to identify the relevance of the project to the NHS as well as health care in general. This will be one of the first sections that is read by a reviewer, so first impressions are important. Don't exceed any word limit that is specified. Try to write in a jargon-free style, such that any health service professional would be easily able to understand the substance of your proposal and be able to appreciate its relevance. The summary should be brief, clear and informative, giving a flavour of what is intended and why.

Literature review

Provide a concise summary of the existing state of knowledge in the project field. The presence of relevant and recent literature in your review will reassure a specialist reviewer that you know what you are talking about. The absence of such literature will not impress the reviewer and could be potentially quite damning. Use the literature to show that there is a gap to be filled, a next step to be taken, or a concern arising. Your aim is to lead the reader in a continuous, logical fashion towards the conclusion you have reached: that this is work that needs to be done, with aims as stated and in the way you have proposed.

Problem statement	Give two to three sentences that state the existing problem and the purpose of the study. Identify what major problems or issues your study is addressing. After reading a problem statement the reviewer should have an idea of why you wish to conduct your study. Problem statements are often seen as separate to research objectives and elaborate on how the study will be conducted.
Hypothesis or research question	State your prediction or question. Be clear and focused. It may be appropriate to pose several related research questions rather than attempt to roll them all into one complex question. If you are making predictions, be clear whether you are making a one-tailed or two-tailed hypothesis (see Chapter 9).
Population	Define the population for whom the results are generalizable as specifically as possible. Make sure you are absolutely clear whether the method you have chosen to obtain a research sample will allow you to make generalizations to a wider population. Beware of assuming wider implications for your research than is actually warranted. You may need formal statistical advice on this for some proposals.
Definition of terms	Define any terms that will be used in the study. Be explicit as to how the term is to be employed in the context of the study. Make it clear whether you are following definitions that are generally accepted in your profession or whether you have devised new or special definitions for the purpose of your study.
Assumptions	Provide the reader with any assumptions that have been made about participant availability, the reliability or validity of measurement tools and the general practicalities of the project. Be honest! Everyone knows that research is not a perfect practice and there are bound to be some limitations to your study, particularly if it is a student project. Common assumptions and limitations centre on the number of participants you think you can recruit into the study within the proposed time-scale.
Research design/ method	Describe the kind of research design and/or method that is to be employed to test the hypothesis or answer the research question(s) in the study (see Chapter 3). In projects that have a predominantly quantitative or experimental nature you can be very explicit about your research design or method. You will be able to specify such things as how many groups of participants you will have, and what will be measured or manipulated. With more qualitative research styles such as ethnography you may be resistant to prespecifying details of the project. The design and maybe the theoretical framework will emerge during the project. Proposals for this type of work must convince the reader that the researcher has a real need (and right) to do this type of research. Whatever the research style, you will need to convince the reader that you are capable of carrying out the proposed methods.

Measurement device/ instrumentation

Describe the tools that will be used to collect the relevant data for your study. Indicate the rationale for selecting them and also any shortcomings they may show which could have implications for the study. It may be appropriate to include samples of the selected tools as appendices, e.g. questionnaires, interview schedules and data collection sheets. Think carefully about what equipment or measurement tools you can legitimately or easily acquire in order to conduct your study. Does your department have equipment you can borrow? Will you need to ask for funding in order to obtain the necessary equipment? Will you need to arrange special insurance in order to use the equipment? If you wish to use a standardized assessment or a commonly used questionnaire, do you have copyright permission? If you intend to design your own data collection tools what steps will you take to ensure their reliability and validity (see Chapter 8)?

Sample selection

Indicate the size of the sample you will use, describe exactly how you will select the sample for the study and the numbers of participants you will use. Identify any anonymity or confidentiality issues and indicate how you will address them. You need to inform the reader of who the sample population will be, including criteria for inclusion into the sample. While you need to be explicit in your inclusion criteria, you also need to be realistic. Although the size of the sample is important, an accurate number of participants required cannot always be given. This is because it is often difficult to predict exactly how many people will agree to take part, qualify to take part and be available to take part within the set time-scale, or how many will begin to take part but drop out.

The number of people agreeing to take part may be influenced by the nature of the study. Few people will volunteer for a study that involves noxious conditions such as inducement of pain! If you are hoping to conduct statistical analyses then consult statistical books and experts for the minimum number of people required to run a particular test successfully. You will need to be explicit about how the participants will be recruited and by whom. If you are a student then you will often be required to ask a qualified person to recruit participants on your behalf. You will need to outline how the study will protect participants from experiencing physical or psychological harm. You also need to address how you will prevent the information gathered from participants being accessed by inappropriate people.

Data collection and procedure

Describe in detail exactly how you plan to carry out the research study. It is often reassuring to the reader if you have carried out some previous work to prepare the ground for the study. This may have been part of an earlier study or project that inspired you to develop the research further. Or you might have carried out specific pilot work, perhaps to demonstrate the feasibility of what you are now proposing. Any necessary permissions for access, co-operation or involvement will have to be negotiated prior to presenting the proposal, and statements concerning such permissions should be included in this section (possibly with documented evidence such as confirmation letters).

Data analysis

Give an indication of the methods that will be used to analyse the data collected. This could be general and broad, e.g. data will be analysed by hand and presented descriptively, or more specific, e.g. data will be entered into a computer software package and analysed for statistical significance. Aim to convince the reader that you have thought through the issues. Avoid giving the impression that you are going to gather the data and then think about the analysis afterwards or that you will simply subject the data to a huge number of unspecified analyses. You should indicate the nature and extent of any computer support needed, and how the need will be met.

Time-scale

Give a brief project timetable indicating when each stage of the project will begin and end. The time-scale of a project obviously influences the feasibility and finances of a study, so consider this section carefully. You cannot always be exact in your time predictions because all sorts of unforeseen circumstances will crop up which may delay completion. The unpredictability of research has lead some such as Hicks (1995) to argue that it is probably better to be pessimistic rather than optimistic about time-scales. If you can draw a chart showing the sequence and timing of the main events, this will help to give an overall idea of the project.

Armstrong, Calnan and Grace (1990) argue that research time can be divided into thirds: one third for planning and getting ready, one third for actual data collection and the last third for analysis and writing up. This is likely to differ, however, depending on the nature of your research. It is not unusual in more qualitative studies for the researcher to be analysing and writing up while they are collecting data and for that analysis to influence the data collection. Whatever the nature of the study the details of a timetable are usually in months.

Example of information given about time-scale:
Stage 1: Questionnaire postal survey
Development and pilot: two months
Data collection: four months
Data analysis: two months

Stage 2: Visits to individual departments in order to conduct structured non-participant observations, analysis of patient records and structured interviews.
Development and pilot: two months
Data collection: nine months
Data analysis: three months

Stage 3: Write up and dissemination of results: two months

Costings and resources   Give an estimated total cost of your project. If you are seeking funding you will be required to provide a detailed breakdown of costings in order to justify the total amount asked for. Be prepared to attach costing estimates from manufacturers for any specific or unusual equipment you are requesting. Spell out the financial implications; these may differ depending on whether you are a student or a qualified therapist. Students will probably need to consider the following costs:

1. Photocopying questionnaires, assessment scales or a second copy of your thesis.
2. Printing a draft and final version of the thesis; this may include paying someone to type it for you.
3. Binding the final draft of your thesis. You will often be required to provide a hardbound copy of your thesis, which will have cost implications; shop around.
4. Telephone calls to arrange meetings, discuss ideas, thank participants and seek help.
5. Travel to place(s) of data collection. There is a usually a lot of travel involved in interviewing people at home or multicentre studies.
6. Stationery, such as letters and envelopes and stamps for posting letters and questionnaires. Don't forget that the cost of this may double or triple if you send reply paid envelopes and follow up non-returned questionnaires.

Qualified therapists will need to consider all of the above, but in addition will probably need to focus in some detail on salaries that are going to be paid to the researchers or data collectors (see Chapter 16 for more detail).

References   You may be required to give a reference list for all the authors you have referred to in your literature review or background section. Be sure you only include those references that you have specifically mentioned in your proposal and that are central to your research topic or methodology. Your references should be as recent as possible and preferably from learned or academic journals of high standing. Make sure you use a consistent referencing style throughout your reference section. Common referencing styles for therapists are the Harvard or Vancouver systems (see Chapter 17).

General points   Check that you have completed all the sections adequately. Look for coherence of the aim, method and analysis. The method, together with the analysis, should enable you to answer the questions or predictions stated in your aims. Common problems with proposals are that the method stated answers a different question to that postulated. Try to word the proposal precisely so that the reviewer does not have to waste time reading irrelevant information or space-filling waffle. A good proposal is worded to convince the reviewer that the proposed research merits approval, so try to keep a logical flow of reasoning.

Where guidelines are sent with research proposal forms it is wise to read and adhere to them carefully. When applying for research funding, many a proposal has been thrown out before serious consideration, simply because guidelines have been ignored. If you are in competition for funding or other approval it makes sense to be ultra-careful and professional in your submission.

In the current climate of research, interprofessional collaboration is highly favoured by funding agencies. Collaboration is encouraged in order to avoid research that is biased or narrow in focus, methodology and purpose. The involvement of 'consumers' or 'stakeholders' such as patients, support groups and special interest groups are also gaining importance and is worthwhile considering, depending on the nature of your project (Bury, 1996). Consumers can help you ascertain whether your project is worthwhile, realistic or likely to attract potential participants. Think about the possibilities of getting other people to work with you on your project. Are there clients, patients, support groups, therapists, doctors, engineers, physiologists, psychologists or sociologists who might have an interest in your research topic? If you can identify any interested parties give them a copy of your proposal and see if they are willing to work with you.

EXERCISE

The initial steps or thoughts can be critical in influencing the structure and flow of your proposal. Use the following four steps to help get you started.

Step 1: Write down up to five sentences that accurately reflect your basic area of research interest. For example:

- The subject I am interested in is respiratory diseases.
- I am interested in children with asthma – particularly children with asthma after exercise.
- I would like to find out what level of exercise causes exercise-induced asthma.

Step 2: Ask yourself up to five questions about your identified research topic. For example:
- What work has already been done?
- What age children am I interested in studying?

Step 3: Swap your paper over with up to three of your friends or colleagues. Get them to write down five more questions either in response to your questions or to the research topic identified in step 1. For example:
- Where would you find the subjects?
- How would you define asthma?
- Is it ethical to give people an asthma attack simply for research purposes?

Step 4: In the light of the answers to the questions in steps 2 and 3: (i) develop your research question; and (ii) make a start at answering the who? what? when? where? why? questions in Table 15.1.

Good proposals and bad proposals

Proposals may be rejected or fail to get funding for several reasons. The proposal may not relate to the stated research objectives, strategies or interest of the funding agency. The results of the study may be of little interest to the wider research community. The proposal may poorly written. Finally, the proposal may be fine but the call for proposals is simply oversubscribed.

If the proposal does not relate to the stated research objectives, strategies or interests of one particular funding agency it may well be accepted by another funding agency that has more interest in the chosen research topic. If a proposal is rejected because the results will be of little interest to a wider community then the researcher may do one of two things. He or she may rewrite the literature review and problem statements in order to convince readers that there is a real need to know the results of such a study, or he or she may question whether the research really does need doing.

A poorly written proposal may be sloppy, unrealistic, biased or ill-defined. A sloppy proposal has ignored guidelines, omitted information or failed to present the information in an easily readable and understandable format. An unrealistic project is one that cannot be achieved with the time and resources available. The research personnel may not have sufficient skills to conduct the research. The project may propose to do something that is not actually research or the methodology may be inappropriate to the project. A biased proposal may be one where the researchers have an ideological stance that makes it clear what the results will be before the study has even been conducted. A proposal may also be biased if the researchers have not considered all the appropriate literature or evidence. An ill-defined proposal is one where the research objectives are not clear, the problem statements or research questions are vague or absent or there is no clear theory base or conceptual framework.

EXERCISE

Critiquing a research proposal
Practising reviewing and critiquing other people's research proposals is a good way of finding out what makes a proposal good or bad. Apply what you learn to your own or your colleagues' proposals, and critically evaluate them before submission! Read the proposal in Figure 15.1 carefully. Précis the content of the proposal in five sentences and answer the following questions:

1. Is the proposal easy to understand and summarize?
2. Is adequate information given under each heading?
3. What is the research question or hypothesis; is it easily identifiable?
4. Will the results from the method answer the research question or hypothesis?
5. Do you think the project is achievable?
6. Does the background adequately set the scene for the research project?
7. Would a funding agency outside of the researcher's place of work be interested in funding the research?

Key points

1. A research proposal is an organized plan or statement of intent.
2. Writing a proposal provides a purpose and a measure of accountability.

This proposal is based on work conducted at the Southampton School of Occupational Therapy and Physiotherapy. See Seale, J., Gallagher, C. and Grisbrooke, J. (1996). Fieldwork educator training: design and evaluation of an educational package. *British Journal of Occupational Therapy*, **59**, 11, 529–534.

Title: Clinical/fieldwork supervisor training

Name of investigators: Jani Grisbrooke, Crissi Gallagher and Jane Seale

Summary
During the three years of the Occupational Therapy and Physiotherapy BSc (Hons) course at the School of Occupational Therapy and Physiotherapy at Southampton University, students spend 38 weeks in clinical settings under the supervision of practising therapists. While students are on placement they are enabled to connect theory to practice and learn to work with patients and therapists. The role of a supervisor is to: (1) develop the student professionally; and (2) judge the student's performance, declare any lack of proficiency and offer requisite help. The supervisor's judgement in terms of student grading effects the final honours classification. Thus, training for these supervisors in methods of assessment is crucial to the course. This project aims to develop an educational package which will: (1) offer supervisors a consistent approach to student assessment; and (2) measure the reliability of student performance gradings. The package will be based on a number of case studies of students functioning at various levels of professional ability, which supervisors will practise grading using assessment forms devised by the school. The range of grades given by supervisors will be analysed.

Background
Clinical/fieldwork education plays a key role within the educational programme of occupational therapy and physiotherapy students. The School believes that clinical/fieldwork is fundamental to the development of students into critical and analytical practitioners capable of reflective practice (1). Each of the two professional bodies (College of Occupational Therapists and the Chartered Society of Physiotherapists) requires students to spend a minimum of 1000 hours in the clinical field. The School devotes 38 (out of 112) weeks of the course to clinical/fieldwork placements. The placements are divided into five blocks (A–E) of varying length, throughout the three years. Because the part played by clinical/fieldwork is so important to the whole scheme of professional education it is appropriate that assessment of clinical/fieldwork is included in the final honours classification. The time that our students have in clinical settings is spent under the tuition of practising therapists. Those therapists, as supervisors, have two distinct roles: (1) to develop the student professionally; and (2) to judge the student's performance. For each placement the student is assessed by their supervisor using assessment forms devised by the School. The assessment is criterion-referenced, with the criteria reflecting the aims of each placement and the developmental nature of the clinical/fieldwork education programme. Each of the five placements has an associated assessment form. Students can be graded from A to Fail.

   The move from diploma to degree courses, along with the contribution of clinical/fieldwork to the final honours degrees, has led to an increased recognition of the importance of the role of supervisors in the assessment of clinical practice. This recognition has led to an increasing focus on the preparation of therapists to assume the critical role of supervisor.

Literature review
A number of surveys have been conducted in order to identify the needs of supervisors. Assessment of students emerges as a high priority in most of them (2). Both professional bodies have identified the importance of training for supervisors. The CSP, for example, distinguishes between two types of training programme: type A programmes, which deal with teaching skills, assessment methodologies, feedback, educational theories and teaching and learning styles; and type B programmes, which deal with course details, clarification of roles and specific supervision skills (3). The School has a commitment to providing both types of training to supervisors who teach our students on placement (4). In order to secure standardization of assessment the School has identified a need for supervisors to receive training about general assessment principles and about using the specific assessment forms designed by the School to grade student performance on placement.

Problem statement
The importance of the supervisor's role in the assessment of clinical practice has increased with the recognition of its contribution to the classification of honours degrees. Surveys of supervisors' educational needs highlight a demand for training in assessment techniques. The purpose of this study is to develop an educational package that can be used in the training of supervisors to reliably use the School assessment forms.

Research question
Can the use of a case-study-based educational package help supervisors reliably grade student performance?

Population
Occupational therapy and physiotherapy supervisors who attend briefing sessions for placement C and D at the School.

Definitions
Supervisor – a therapist who undertakes the teaching and assessment of a student for a whole clinical/fieldwork placement.

Assumptions and limitations
The results of this study will only show whether supervisors have been successfully trained to assess students at Southampton University.

Research design
A survey of 100–150 clinical/fieldwork supervisors.

Measurement device/instrumentation
Clinical Placement Assessment form.

Selection of participants
1. *Briefing session:* Around 100–150 supervisors who attend briefing sessions for placement C and D. Therapists have 'volunteered' to be supervisors and are not selected in any way. Attendance at the briefing session is a requirement that has to be met by all supervisors before the School places a student in the care of a supervisor. Supervisors will be informed that the content of the briefing sessions will include some data collection.
2. *Rating exercise:* Ten volunteer school staff (excluding project team) will be involved in rating the case studies. The numbers of occupational therapists and physiotherapists will be equal.

Collection of data
1. *Creation of case studies:* A set of 10 case studies will be devised that illustrate a wide range of student competencies which can be assessed using the assessment form devised by the School. Together the case studies should enable the whole range of grades to be used. It is felt that these case studies must be based on an understanding of how experienced therapists reason about their practice, and therefore the help of an experienced therapist would be sought in the creation of the case studies.
2. *School rating exercise:* Once the case studies have been devised, 10 School staff will be asked to use the assessment form to grade the student described in each case. The staff will be asked to grade the same cases twice (with a suitable gap in the middle) in order to check test–retest reliability. The five case studies that produce the most discrepancy in grading will be discarded.
3. *Briefing exercise with supervisors:* For each briefing session that the School has to run, the session leader will present the supervisors with the five case studies. The group will be introduced to the assessment form and then asked to use the form to grade the student presented in each case study.

Analysis of data
1. *Rating exercise:* The kappa test statistic will be used to analyse test–retest reliability. This test will be run using the statistical package SPSS.
2. *Briefing exercise:* The grade that each supervisor gives for each case study will be compared with the expected grade in order to calculate the percentage of agreement between the supervisors and expected grades. This descriptive analysis will be run using the statistical package SPSS.

Time-scale
1. Development of case studies: Two months; 2. rating exercise: one month; 3. briefing exercise: three months; 4. data analysis: one month; 5. write up: two months.

Costings
Therapists' time: £4923; clerical support: £1829; materials: £200.

References
1. Southampton School of Occupational Therapy and Physiotherapy (1993). BSc (Hons) in Occupational Therapy and BSc (Hons) in Physiotherapy. Validation document.
2. Chartered Society of Physiotherapy Clinical Education Working Party (1994). Guidelines for good practice for the education of clinical educators. *Physiotherapy*, **80**, 299–230.
3. Walker, E.M. and Openshaw, S. (1994). Educational needs as perceived by clinical supervisors. *Physiotherapy*, **80**, 424–431.
4. Southampton School of Occupational Therapy and Physiotherapy (1994). *Clinical/Fieldwork Education Supervisors' Handbook.*

Figure 15.1   Sample proposal.

3. Supervisors, funding agencies and ethical committees might read your proposal.
4. Criteria such as value and appropriateness might be used to judge your proposal.
5. The tasks involved in writing a research proposal range from conducting a literature review to completing a proposal form.
6. When completing a proposal form be coherent, follow guidelines and collaborate with stakeholders.
7. Proposals get rejected because they do not relate to the interests of the funding agency, are of little interest to the wider community, are poorly written or are responding to a call for proposals that is oversubscribed.
8. A poorly written proposal is sloppy, unrealistic, biased and ill-defined.

References

Armstrong, D., Calnan, M. and Grace, J. (1990). *Research Methods for General Practitioners*. Oxford Medical Publications.

Bury, T. (1996). *Introduction to Research*. Chartered Society of Physiotherapy.

Currier, D. (1990). *Elements of Research in Physical Therapy*, 3rd Edn. Williams and Wilkins.

Hicks, C.M. (1995). *Research for Physiotherapists: Project Design and Analysis*, 2nd Edn. Churchill Livingstone.

Robson, C. (1993). *Real World Research: A Resource for Social Scientists and Practitioner-Researchers*. Blackwell.

Complementary reading

Drummond, A. (1996). *Research Methods for Therapists*. Chapman & Hall. Chapter 1, Section 5: Writing a protocol.

French, S. (1993). *Practical Research: A Guide for Therapists*. Butterworth-Heinemann. Chapter 4: Writing a research proposal.

Payton, O. (1988). *Research: The Validation of Clinical Practice*, 2nd Edn. F.A. Davis Company. Appendix A: Outline for writing a research protocol. Appendix B: Reconstructed protocol.

Costing your research project and seeking funds

The cost of undertaking research

The cost of undertaking research varies dramatically depending on the type of research project being undertaken. A low key in-house project will accrue only slight cost but a multicentre, large cohort, longitudinal study involving many researchers, perhaps expensive drugs or assessment equipment and complex analysis will cost many tens or hundreds of thousands of pounds. Even the simplest of student projects will incur some cost and this should be taken into consideration when deciding whether a project is feasible. Some costs, such as buying in statistical advice and photocopying the hundreds of sheets of paper that comprise your questionnaires, are obvious. However, there are many hidden costs that are not always obvious to a new researcher which also need to be taken into account. The next section looks at some of the things you need to consider when costing a research project. Although this looks specifically from the UK perspective, the principles can be applied similarly to other countries.

Personnel costs

Personnel costs include costs for researchers, supervisors, secretarial and administrative support, expert advice and data preparation and entry, plus steering group and participant costs.

Researcher costs include the salary of the researcher and any costs associated with advertising the post. If you are the researcher it may also include the cost of buying out your time or buying in someone to job-share. When costing for a researcher's salary you need to indicate at what scale you want to employ the person and give a breakdown of annual costs such as National Insurance contributions and super-annuation. You may need to include incremental or inflationary rises if the project is going to run for more than a year. It is accepted that short-term contract researchers are paid slightly more than long-term employed staff.

If the researcher is inexperienced in research, some supervision will be necessary from someone with more experience. If the supervision amounts to a regular session of, say, half a day per week, then the cost of the supervision will need to be included.

Most research projects will require a degree of basic administration, ranging from photocopying and stuffing questionnaires into envelopes to arranging appointments for research participants and transcribing interview data. These sorts of jobs are suited to administrative assistance rather than to researcher or therapist time. Transcribing taped interviews is an expert skill. Some secretaries are happy to do this but you may need to buy in specialist assistance, which is expensive but can make the data analysis task very much easier.

Most universities will have a statistics department that you can tap into for expert statistical advice. Some departments offer an hour of free advice then charge by the hour, day or project. Check with your local department. You will need to discuss with your statistician whether you just need advice on the right statistical test to use and what data should be collected or whether you need much more involvement from them in the analysis and interpretation of data. Statisticians are highly qualified and will expect reasonable remuneration, so it is vital not to leave this out of your costing calculation.

Similarly, you may need to buy in some software support for any computer package you are using. Do not forget other expert advice that may be needed. For example, if you are conducting a blinded trial into the efficacy of a particular intervention for patients with acute low back pain, you may need to pay therapists to undertake the assessments of the patients you are treating, so as to ensure there is no bias in the data collected. If training is required to ensure reliability of the assessment, then you will need to add in the training costs also.

Coding questionnaire data and entering them into a data analysis package on the computer is a monotonous and time-consuming task. It is also a skilled job, requiring accuracy in both coding and inputting skills. If you have a lot of data it may be cost- and time-effective to send the work out to an agency skilled in this area. Some universities can provide this service (often postgraduate students paying their way through PhD studies) or commercial agencies may be contacted through the 'Phone Book'.

It is usual for a steering group to meet regularly during the course of a research project (see Chapter 13). You will need to consider the cost of travel to the meetings, hiring of a meeting room, refreshments, photocopying and postage of materials for the meeting and any fee or honorarium for the participants.

The participants or subjects are the most important personnel in your project, for without them there can be no project! It will almost certainly cost some money to recruit and include them. Some subjects will need to be recruited through advertisements that have to be paid for. Where research could cause some discomfort, for example where people volunteer to have muscle or skin biopsies, or where there may be an element of psychological stress, a payment may be made. Many universities and NHS Trusts will have policies regarding payment of subjects, so it is wise to consult about this. You may feel that participants should be remunerated for their expertise. For example, if your project includes a focus group looking at the experiences of disabled people in hospital you may feel you want to pay participants for their time and knowledge. Check with participants that any payment does not have an adverse impact on any benefits they receive. Even if you are not paying people for their participation you may need to reimburse them for any loss of earnings which they incur. Many projects rely on volunteers but even then there may be costs. You need to consider travel expenses and hidden costs such as child care or carer cover. Do not forget the cost of any refreshments, parking or room hire. If your participants are NHS patients you may need to consider the extra cost of your research to the NHS (see separating the cost of research from NHS costs later in this chapter).

Equipment

Equipment that you may need to budget for includes computer hardware and software, measurement and collection tools and consumables.

These days it is almost impossible to undertake research without a computer. You will need it for generating data collection sheets or questionnaires, writing letters to the steering group and participants, number crunching the data and producing reports and papers. A computer linked into the 'Web' via a modem will open up a vista of information via the Internet and allow you to communicate with experts all over the world using e-mail. If you do not have easy access to a suitable computer then you will need to add the cost of this, a suitable printer and appropriate software to your shopping list, together with any necessary training and support.

Look around for the most appropriate software for your research. You will need a word processing package and some statistical software or a spreadsheet package for data analysis. A graphics package will make light work of figures and tables for the final report and presentations. If you are working at a university or health service unit check with the computing services or IT department as they often have access to site licences or can give you a good deal on purchasing both hardware and software. Do not forget to purchase a copious number of floppy disks so that you can keep back-up copies of your work in different safe places. A lockable disk box and filing cabinet or drawer is vital for storing your data, not only to prevent them from getting lost but also to assure the local ethics committee that confidential data are being stored securely.

Research equipment may range from a simple goniometer to an expensive custom-built gait analysis rig. Ensure that the equipment is going to be available before you start the project. Do not forget that there may be a delay between ordering and delivery of specialist equipment due to manufacturing processes.

One-to-one interviews may be recorded adequately using a standard cassette recorder. However, when recording a number of people in a focus group, better results are obtained using specialist, higher quality, equipment and a multi-directional microphone. Although tapes may be transcribed using a standard cassette recorder it is less time consuming and less strain on the tape to use a proper transcriber with a foot switch for winding and rewinding the tape. Secretaries will appreciate the use of a proper commercial transcribing machine and this should be considered in the project costings where appropriate. Use a new audio tape for each interview if possible, as this allows for more than one transcriber, to speed up the data preparation process. It also prevents getting muddled between subjects. The authors do not recommend the use of audio tapes any longer than C90, as longer ones tend to be very thin and stretchy, causing problems with playback and possible snapping.

It is easy to forget consumables like tissues, ultrasound gel, splinting materials and videotapes which soon add up to a considerable sum. Write down the methodology of your research project in the most detail you possibly can and then highlight all the equipment and consumables you intend to use. Multiply these by the number of participants, including some extra for piloting and familiarization with the process and techniques you will be using. This will give you an idea of how much you will need. Check ordering and delivery times to ensure you are not left having to cancel experiments or other data collection due to the absence of a simple piece of equipment.

Running costs

Running costs include telephone, stationery, postage, photocopying and travel costs. Calculate telephone costs based on expected usage. Will you be using the phone infrequently just to order equipment or check that steering group members can make a meeting? Or will you be using it to arrange appointments for participants? Or will you be a heavy user, undertaking telephone interviews with many participants? Your workplace may be happy to absorb the costs if they are light but you will certainly need to cost for heavy usage.

Cost for the paper used in questionnaire design and production, data collection sheets, letters and information sheets to participants, hand-outs and reports to steering group members, executive summaries to interested parties and final reports to key players or the commissioners of your research. The cost of the final report may be offset by charging for copies sent to other interested parties, although you will need to clear this with your workplace and any commissioners or funders of your research. If you are sending out questionnaires remember to cost for large enough envelopes, not forgetting the cost of the return envelope too. You will need files for keeping your data and draft reports, overhead projector acetates and pens for presentations and ink cartridges for your printer.

Remember to cost for outward and return paid postage for postal questionnaires. Weigh an envelope with all its enclosures as you may need to cost for more than a standard stamp. Project reports are weighty bundles and will cost more for postage. If your research is to involve a lot of postage, talk to your workplace to arrange franking for outgoing post and a licence for prepaid returned post. It is easier to settle an invoice than lick hundreds of stamps!

It is easy to photocopy and just as easy to forget the cost of each sheet. Calculate the amount of copying carefully, including the final report and executive summary, if appropriate, to add into your final costings.

Calculate the mileage or public transport costs involved in travelling to your subjects, your subjects travelling to you (if appropriate), travel to steering groups and travel to conferences (if appropriate).

Reporting back

In costing for reporting back you will need to take into account report production and distribution, feedback workshops and conference attendance. Every research project has a report whether it is one copy of your dissertation for the examiners or many copies for the commissioners of a piece of work and the general public (see Chapter 19). A dissertation will probably need to be bound in some way (ask your examining university) and this may cost a few pence for a ring binder or several pounds for book binding. Larger print runs will involve the cost of printing and any artwork or designer's fees for illustrations, as well as the cost of the paper and card covers or other binding. Although it may be possible to recoup some of this cost with sales of your report, you will need to pay the money 'up front' to the printer. Remember to add in the cost of packing (often a large padded envelope will do) and postage for distribution.

If many people have assisted you in your research or are interested in its results, it may be a good idea to hold a conference or workshop to feed back the results. Costs incurred for this include the hire of a conference room, publicity or invitations, secretarial support, refreshments, keynote speaker fees, copies of the executive summary or full report for each delegate and production of any slides or other audio-visual presentation.

Useful research findings should be disseminated and this means attending conferences to give papers or poster presentations and writing papers for academic and professional journals. Costs associated with this include the production of presentation and poster materials, travel and, possibly, overnight accommodation and subsistence. Unless you are very lucky, the preparation of these presentations will have to be done in your own time!

Overheads

Employing researchers and administrative staff incurs overhead costs for the institution where the project is being undertaken. This includes such things as the employer's National Insurance contribution, office accommodation and heating and lighting. The amount of overheads charged varies between institutions and between funding bodies. It often varies between 10% and 50%. Funding bodies often have an

Table 16.1 Example of salary and overhead costing

Scale	Grade	Spine	Salary	NI	Pens.	Subtotal	Total (inc. 40% overheads)	Total for four years
Research Fellow (F/T)	1A	09	18,294	1408	3394	23,096	32,334.4	129,337.6
Secretary (0.5 WTE)	CLE1	07	4059	207	419	4685	6559	26,236

overhead rate above which they will not go. Some funding bodies have negotiated rates with individual institutions. Check with your employing institution and funding body for accurate information (see Table 16.1 for an example).

Working out your budget

When working out the budget for a research project it is important to take a step-by-step approach. Use your research protocol to identify all the potential costs using the above lists as a guide. Highlight the resources, equipment, expertise and running costs that will need to be funded. Contact the finance officer in your workplace to establish any overhead costs. Costs may be reduced by negotiation. For example, you may be able to use existing departmental equipment or facilities after patient treatment hours for conducting clinical research or running-off questionnaires. Some funding bodies will not pay for things that they consider to be standard university or departmental equipment. For example, university staff would find it difficult to justify research grant funding for a computer, although they may be able to obtain specialist software. A clinical department, however, may be able to make a good case for computer hardware to support a research project on the grounds that the appropriate equipment is not standard issue in an NHS therapy department.

Accuracy of budgeting can be vital to the project. If you are applying to a funding body it is likely that the reviewers will look very closely at the costings. It is vital to justify each item on the budget plan in as much depth as possible. Do not expect to use a research grant to re-equip the department or provide extra administrative support for another project. A request for £500 for travel will need to be justified in terms of rate per mile and distance as well as number of trips. Funding bodies have very many demands on their limited funds and 'guesstimation' is not good enough. It looks very poor if the methodology does not marry up with the budget. For example, a proposal that has not accurately identified the number of participants cannot possibly forecast the cost of interview transcription. When funding is so competitive a poorly laid out budget plan can lead to rejection of the whole project for funding, regardless of how pertinent the research question is. It is equally important not to underestimate the costs. A good project may fall to pieces simply because the cost of data preparation and entry was not considered, as the applicant did not realize how much time it would involve and is not able to undertake it himself. Help with putting together a budget plan for your research project is available from NHS Executive Regional Research and Development Offices, local NHS Trust Research Support Units and from academic departments at your local university.

Looking for extra funding

There are hundreds of grant-giving bodies funding everything from science to art, from major international medical drugs trials for cancer to small, single case studies in learning disabilities. Find out what is available. Many of the more prestigious grants come from highly respected organizations such as the Medical Research Council or the Economic and Social Research Council (ESRC). These bodies receive hundreds of applications and if you submit to these or similar bodies you need to know that you are facing stiff competition from some of the most experienced researchers (and proposal writers!) in the country. It is probably true that funding bodies look at the past research experience of the applicant, including their track record in publications and successful grant application. If you are well known in your field it certainly helps with grant application, although it is by no means certain that your project will get funded. A sloppy application will fail regardless of your professional or academic status. However, for less experienced researchers there are many smaller, less well known charities and trusts who are well worth approaching.

The Association of Medical Research Charities produces a handbook each year listing 50 or so medical charities that offer research grants. The handbook gives information about the type of research funded and the level of grants usually awarded. Most are awarded in competition and ask for submission of a protocol and budget plan. Most have a closing date for applications. Some award several times a year, others annually. As a general guide, small grants mean those of up to £10,000 awarded as a one-off payment. Large grants are up to £50,000 per year for three years. Very small grants of a few hundred pounds are well worth applying for, as they may pay for travel or equipment costs. They also give you valuable experience of grant application as well as another successful submission to put on your CV. Other sources of grant information include *The Directory of Grant Making Trusts* and *The Charities Digest*. These are often available in public as well as medical and academic libraries.

Having found out what is available you need to decide where exactly to submit. Look at your research question. If it is condition or pathology specific see if there is a relevant charity to contact. Some funding bodies call for proposals in certain fields so watch the professional and academic press for calls relevant to your proposed area of research. Others have a more general remit and you may submit anything that is encompassed by the frame of reference of the funder. If your research question is therapy specific contact your professional body for details of grants. The Physiotherapy Research Foundation can be contacted through the CSP Research and Development Officer at the Chartered Society of Physiotherapy. This Foundation considers research bids of up to £10,000 and has one call for submissions, currently in February each year. The College of Occupational Therapy offers several small grants each year to assist occupational therapy research (details from COT).

Most grant-awarding bodies will tell you what format they want your submission to take. Many will provide an application form and guidelines for completion. Read and adhere to the guidelines very carefully to ensure that you are making your application to the right body and giving them the information they require. Some funders have two rounds of submission, especially those who receive a large number of applications. An outline proposal is considered first and, if successful, a full proposal is requested. An outline proposal usually consists of a sheet of double-sided A4 that briefly outlines your research question, methodology and sample, together with the experience of the researcher. These are considered and, if the research proposal is felt to warrant closer consideration, a full proposal is requested. A full proposal may consist of a long submission clearly setting out the research question, the background to the research, the need for the investigation and the practicalities of undertaking the project. In effect, the project must be ready to 'get up and go', with all the practical and academic elements of the project fully considered and accounted for. In practice this means working up a full protocol, agreeing any necessary collaboration with clinicians, managers and academics and obtaining ethical approval. This may seem a lot of effort to go to if there is absolutely no certainty of funding and indeed it is.

If your submission is turned down you often receive feedback which you may like to consider before resubmitting your proposal. Check with the funding body as to whether they accept resubmissions or look for another prospective funder. Having proposals rejected for funding is part of a researcher's life. It is very disappointing to have so much hard work flushed away but there cannot be an experienced researcher in the country who has not had to deal with this kind of disappointment. Do not let a disappointment like this prevent you from trying again.

Some funding bodies will ask to interview you prior to making a decision about your proposal. This is more common in submissions where the research will lead to the researcher gaining a higher degree. The process is similar to a job interview with short-listing for interview following from consideration of the application. Again, most applications are submitted on standard forms. If you are called for interview be prepared to give a short presentation about your research idea and ensure that you will be able to answer questions about both the practical and academic elements of the research.

Grant-awarding bodies will be looking for the following in your application:

1. A pertinent research question.
2. Research that will benefit the aims of the funding body, e.g. will be of benefit to the NHS or to people with stroke etc.
3. A well considered ethical approach.
4. A 'do-able' methodology.
5. Evidence of collaboration with clinicians, academics and managers where appropriate.
6. Some insight into any possible limitations or pitfalls.
7. An experienced researcher or supervision by an experienced researcher.

8. Realistic budget that matches the methodology and adheres to funder's guidelines.
9. Potentially publishable, generalizable results.

Seeking small sums

It is not always necessary to go to major funding bodies to gain financial assistance for your research. If you are working in a hospital take your research proposal to your line manager and the management board (Trust board in the NHS). Some hospitals have trust or endowment funds that can be tapped for small amounts. The League of Friends may be willing to purchase equipment needed for the research. It is also worth approaching commercial organizations such as drug or equipment companies for support. It is wise to do this through your hospital management board or research support unit as they may have protocols for working with commercial enterprises.

Separating the cost of research from NHS costs

If you are conducting research on NHS staff or patients you need to be aware of the recent funding changes. It may seem easy to call a patient back for another appointment just to gather data for your research but every intervention has a cost and it is not appropriate or indeed allowable for NHS patient costs to subsidize NHS research and development activity. The Culyer Report (1994) recommended the split of patient and research costs and from 1998 the full recommendations will come into play (NHSE, 1997). Each Trust will have to negotiate for R&D funds from the NHSE. Researchers may then bid for these monies to cover the cost of extra patient appointments, consumables such as X-rays and other extra materials necessary for the research. For example, researchers could bid for funds to cover the cost of more expensive drugs in a comparative trial. Researcher costs will be expected to be paid for by other funds such as charities and commercial or research grants. Local arrangements regarding this research and development levy are available from individual NHS Trusts.

Training awards

There are funds available to assist therapists seeking higher degrees. These include research-based Masters degrees, MPhil/PhD studentships and postdoctoral fellowships. Full studentships, funding your salary, fees and research costs for the duration of your degree (usually three years for a PhD), are highly competitive and are available through NHSE regions, the Medical Research Council and some charitable bodies and councils. In most cases you will be competing against medics and other medical scientists and clinicians not just therapists. Part funding can be obtained from departmental training budgets in your workplace, small studentship grants offered by academic departments in universities and educational grants from professional bodies. Many people undertake part-time studies and work to pay their way. Occasionally an experienced researcher may be successful in a grant application for a project that requires a research assistant who can gain a higher degree through that project. Contact your local university departments to let them know you would be interested if any of these opportunities come up.

Hints for submitting a successful application

1. Submit to the right place at the right time.
2. Work up outline proposals by identifying research questions and keeping up to date with the literature, policy and practice in your chosen area so that you can put a proposal together quickly when a call is published; often there is little time between the call and the submission date.
3. Keep to the funder's guidelines for application.
4. If you are new to research consider collaboration with an expert in the field or someone with a track record in successful grant applications.

Key points

1. All research has a monetary cost ranging from hundreds of thousands of pounds for a multi-centre study to an insignificant amount to cover photocopying costs for a small in-house project.
2. Project costs accrue from employing personnel, computing requirements, equipment, consumables, travel, reimbursement of participants' costs, production of the final report and overheads.
3. Calculate an accurate budget accounting for all possible costs. Assistance can be obtained from the finance officers of academic institutions, local NHS Research and Support Units, NHS Executive Regional Research and Development Offices and other funding bodies.
4. Submitting applications for funding to grant-giving bodies is highly competitive. Pay attention to the remit of the body, the required submission format and any guidelines for its completion.
5. The cost of research in the National Health Service must now be separated from NHS patient and clinical costs.
6. Training awards are available for therapists wishing to undertake research towards a higher degree.

References

AMRC (1996). *The Association of Medical Research Charities Handbook 1996–1997.* AMRC.

NHS Executive (1997). Meeting patient care costs associated with R&D in the NHS: detailed guidance. EL(97)77. Department of Health, Leeds.

The Culyer Report (1994). *Supporting Research and Development in the NHS. A Report to the Minister of Health.* HMSO.

The Family Welfare Association (1995). *The Charities Digest*, 101st Edn. The Family Welfare Association.

Villemur, A. (1995). *The Directory of Grant Making Trusts.* CAF.

Complementary reading

Chartered Society of Physiotherapy (1996). *Introduction to Research.* CSP Education Department.

Phillips, E.M. and Pugh, D. S. (1994). *How to Get a PhD: A Handbook for Students and Their Supervisors.* Open University Press.

17 Writing up your research: presenting your results

The task of communication

Communicating the results of a study is an important part of the whole research process (Drummond, 1996) and yet it is, for most of us, the hardest part. Part of what makes it so hard is that we 'suddenly' have to get back in touch with the purpose of the research study in order to work out whether we have found what we expected to find. When we are data collecting it is easy to 'forget' why we are collecting the data and just get caught up in the flow and process of getting the results.

In writing up the results of a research project, we often have to ask ourselves some very searching questions. Questions such as: Did I use the right methodology? Can I make sense of the data? Was this study worth doing after all? Sometimes the answers to these questions are painful ones and this can make the writing up process a difficult one. But it is not always doom and gloom. Writing up a research project can be a very creative experience. If you are able to get in 'control' of the data then you can use them to support your ideas, develop new theories and influence thinking and practice. In this chapter we will cover what should go in a complete research report, before looking in more detail at the results section of a report.

Compiling a standard research report

The structure of your research report will reflect the various stages of the data project and may use the following headings: title, abstract, introduction, method, results, discussion, conclusion, references and appendices. The different sections of your report should be linked in a clear and concise manner. What will help you link the sections is the research question. Keep going back to it and ask yourself if you are answering that question. You are probably going to be judged on how well your report answered the question you posed yourself. The introduction and discussion are both weighty sections of a research report that reviewers will be inspecting carefully to assess the extent to which you understand the research process in general and the full implications of your own research question.

Title page

The title should give a clear and concise indication of the nature of the project. Whatever the title is, it should be accurate, informative and not too long. If you are conducting an experimental project you may find it useful to construct a title from the relationship predicted in your hypothesis (Hicks, 1995).

Abstract

An abstract is a summary of your project and should be roughly 150 words. A reader should be able to tell from the abstract enough about the project to decide whether it is interesting/relevant and therefore whether to spend time reading the full report. Make sure that the abstract can be fully understood without reference to any other part of the write up. An abstract should include the aim or question of the research, methods used and a brief indication of the main findings and their implications. Although an abstract appears at the beginning of the report most people find it best to write it up after they have written the rest of the report.

Introduction

The introduction will set the scene to your project, and should give enough background information to place it in context and provide a theoretical frame of reference. An introduction begins with general statements about the topic and then moves to a critical discussion of the literature that has a specific relevance to your question. In providing a theoretical framework you will need to refer to the work of others.

> **Example:** Bloggs (1979) found that 43% of university lecturers reported feelings of indifference to exercise, while Bloggette (1985) found that 60% of university lecturers in her sample reported positive attitudes to exercise. The reasons for this discrepancy may be due to the different measurement techniques the two researchers used.

Full references to the studies you mention here should be given in the reference section of the report. The introduction should end with a clear statement of what is being investigated and its relevance to clinical practice. Remember an introduction is not a review of all the research ever done on a topic. If your research topic is a little unusual or 'off the beaten track' then you should probably spend some time justifying (through the use of literature) why you think your particular topic needs researching.

Method

In this section you will need to describe the nature of the data collected, who they were collected from and how. You need to ensure sufficient clarity and precision to allow another researcher to replicate your project. A methodology section will need to include information about the number and description of participants, how participants were selected, a description of data collection instruments and apparatus used (bikes, scales, etc.) and a description of the procedure, including how the performance of participants was measured and recorded (see Figure 17.1 for an example). You may also need to describe how you dealt with ethical issues such as informed consent and confidentiality.

The research team decided that it would be useful to survey clinical/ fieldwork educators about their experience of the briefing sessions and how that experience helped them to grade a real student who they supervised on placement. A questionnaire was designed in order to ascertain this information. The questionnaire was three pages long and had four sections:

Section 1: Background information. This section asked for details such as profession, length of supervising experience and nature of previous contacts with students.
Section 2: Experience of briefing sessions. This section asked respondents to evaluate how useful they found the briefing session and elicited opinions as to the critical factors at play when trying to grade a hypothetical student.
Section 3: Grading students on placement. In this section opinions were elicited regarding the critical factors at play when grading a Southshore student at the half-way and completion stages, along with the characteristics that they think are representative of a student who is achieving grades A, B, C, D or Fail.
Section 4: Personal comments. This section invited respondents to make any additional comments about their experience of the briefing sessions and grading Southshore students.

The questionnaire was sent with a covering letter to 70 placement clinical/ fieldwork educators. The covering letter asked respondents to indicate when they returned their questionnaire whether they would be willing to take part in a follow-up interview about their experiences of the briefing session.

Figure 17.1   Example of a method section.

Example: The interviews lasted approximately an hour and were tape-recorded. The interviewees consented to being audio-taped and were aware that the tapes would be stored in a locked filing cabinet during the study and then destroyed six months after the study was completed. The researcher also gave an undertaking that the names of the interviewees would not be divulged in the project report.

It is also important that you justify your methodology. For example, if you chose to interview your subjects, why? What were the advantages of conducting an interview over any other comparable method such as a questionnaire? It may be appropriate to explain small sample sizes and a lack of control groups or any other design feature that one might normally expect from a 'textbook project'. You will also need to address reliability and validity issues.

Results

This section contains the 'facts' of your project. It is usual to begin with more general results and then move to more specific findings. If you have a lot of data you may need to be selective in what you present. You should nonetheless make sure that you present a well-balanced picture. Make sure that everything you include in this section is there to make a point and not merely to pad things out. Charts and tables should be accompanied by a brief written explanation. Make

Table 5. Kappa statistic and mean percentage agreement for the four sections of the assessment form

Statistic	Safety	Interpersonal	Clinical	Management
Kappa	0.89051	0.57092	0.5454	0.56104
Mean % agreement	98.1500	70.8000	65.9500	69.6000

Table 5 shows that the raters were most agreed and reliable for the safety section followed by the interpersonal, management and clinical sections. Overall the case studies appear to elicit moderate test–retest reliability.

Figure 17.2   Presenting results using a table.

sure graphs, charts and tables are numbered and titled (see Figure 17.2 for an example).

If you are using descriptive statistics alone then you may like to remind the reader at the beginning of this section why this is; for example, small subject numbers or not meeting the criteria of a particular statistical test (equal numbers of subjects, normal distribution etc.). If you are using statistical tests then you need to tell the reader which test you used and what p values and levels of significance were achieved. Avoid excessive statistical detail as this may confuse some readers depending on your target audience.

Example: A Spearman's correlation test was applied to test the correlations between different stress parameters and working conditions. A positive correlation was found to exist between staff turnover and intensity of job stress. This was significant at the 5% level ($R_s = 0.734$, $p < 0.05$).

If you have qualitative data then your results section will probably not look conventional. You are likely to have more data than you really know what to do with, so you need to think very carefully about how you present your results. Raw data are not presented in the text but are given in an appendix.

An interesting issue is the extent to which we should interpret results in the results section. For traditional experimental results, researchers are usually quite clear that no description of method or discussion should take place in a results section, only the reporting of results (Currier, 1990). For more qualitative methodologies, such as in-depth interviews, some argue that it makes sense to combine presentation with interpretation (French, 1993).

Discussion and conclusion

The discussion section will interpret and debate your findings as well as place them in a theoretical context by relating them to the research highlighted in the introduction. You may discuss your results in relation to any or all of the following issues: whether the results found were expected and, if not, then possible reasons for their occurrence might be discussed; whether the results confirm findings from other research; and whether the results extend or clarify a particular theory or body of knowledge. You will also need to address any problems with the project that may influence interpretation of the findings, along with implications for clinical practice or further investigations. Keep the discussion relevant and beware of going beyond the scope of your findings in the discussion and making giant leaps or claims that your project cannot support. A more detailed examination of how to write a discussion section will be given in Chapter 18. The conclusion should highlight the main points of the project and emphasize those issues that the reader should remember.

References and appendices

At the end of the report provide a complete list of references. Only list the books and/or articles that you have mentioned in your report. The quality of your work will not be judged on the number of references you cite *per se* but reviewers will be expecting to see evidence of a thorough and up to date literature review. Brodie *et al.* (1994) argue that one of the biggest mistakes is to leave referencing until the end. Although it is a pain to have to keep interrupting writing in order to find references and make sure they are correct, according to Brodie *et al.* it is well worth it, otherwise you are bound to lose some detail and information.

There are two main styles of referencing in therapy research, the Harvard and the Vancouver styles. These styles have rules for how you present references in the text and in the reference list at the end of the report. With the Harvard style, references are indicated in the text by the surname of the author and the year of publication. In the reference list the references are listed by the authors name in alphabetical order.

Example of Harvard referencing:

In text:

While Bloggs (1979) found that 43% of university lecturers reported feelings of indifference to exercise, Bloggette (1985) found that 60% of university lecturers in her sample reported positive attitudes to exercise.

In reference list:

Bloggette, T. (1985). New ways of testing attitudes to exercise in university environments. *Archive of University Medicine*, **65**, 879–885.

Bloggs, J. (1979). University lecturers' attitudes to exercise. *International Journal of Exercise*, **4**, 45–56.

With the Vancouver style, each reference is given a number according to where it appears in the text. When this reference is used, a number appears. In the reference list the references appear in the order that they were mentioned in the text.

> **Example of Vancouver referencing:**
> *In text:*
> Research has revealed mixed results regarding university lecturers' attitudes to exercise.[1,2]
>
> *In reference list:*
> 1. Bloggs, J. (1979). University lecturers' attitudes to exercise. *International Journal of Exercise*, **4**, 45–56.
> 2. Bloggette, T. (1985). New ways of testing attitudes to exercise in university environments. *Archive of University Medicine*, **65**, 879–885.

Detailed information, such as raw data, that would interfere with the flow of text should be located in the appendices which are placed at the end of the report.

The order in which you write the different sections of your report will vary from person to person. Many researchers advise us to begin at the middle of the report and write the method and results sections first. These are thought to be easier to write since they are factual sections, rather than sections that require detailed analysis and interpretation. As these sections take shape they will help to clarify points that need to be raised in the introduction, discussion and conclusions (Drummond, 1996). With more qualitative research, however, the distinction between collecting results and writing them up is less clear. Maykut and Morehouse (1996) note that many writers begin writing early in the process of conducting the research. It is suggested that such early writing helps the researcher to familiarize themselves with the data. These early writings may or may not form part of the final report.

Format and styles of research reports

The format and style of your research report may differ depending on your target audience or whom you are writing the report for. The target audience will influence what sections you include in your report, how long those sections are and what you include in each section.

If you are writing a dissertation or journal article then the format is likely to be similar to the standard research report outlined earlier. In order to impress those reading your dissertation or article you will need to demonstrate detailed critical analysis skills.

If you are writing a report for commissioners or funders of research then you may need to write a short report or executive summary in which you 'cut to the quick' of the results. The skill required here is that of presenting enough information so readers understand the nub of your project without getting lost in a lengthy review or analysis. Some projects will require you to produce interim reports while the study is being done and a final report at the end of the study. The interim reports are likely to focus on methodology and results while the final report may place the results in a context with a literature review and discussion.

With certain kinds of reports you may find that what you include in each section differs slightly to what you would include in a full standard report. For example, it may not be appropriate in a short or interim report to discuss the limitations of the study in the discussion section. In a report written for practitioners you may place a greater emphasis on clinically based literature than on other kinds of literature.

Strauss (1995) suggests that qualitative researchers have three options when presenting their data. They can keep the presentation very abstract and theoretical, they can give very little theoretical commentary, allowing the data to speak for itself, or they can try and find a balance between the two 'extremes'. Strauss suggests that the option the researcher chooses will depend on the purpose of the report and the anticipated readership. If the purpose of the report is to give a sense of reality and provide insight into the world of the 'actors' then the researcher may use lots of illustrative data. If the purpose of the report is to add weight to the researcher's theoretical ideas or commentary then the ratio of interpretation to data will alter accordingly.

A sample results section

The example of a results section given presents the findings of a study designed to investigate the usefulness of an educational package for training clinical fieldwork educators and is based on an article by Seale, Gallagher and Grisbrooke (1996). The educational package consisted of case studies of hypothetical students on clinical placement. The producers of the package were keen to investigate whether the case studies were a useful educational tool in helping clinical fieldwork educators familiarize themselves with the clinical fieldwork assessment criteria. Evaluative data from 300 clinicians were obtained through questionnaires and interviews.

This sample results section will be presented because it is *not* perfect. When you are reading through the sample results section, look at the content of the results and the way they have been presented. Can you identify any areas that the author needs to improve? Compare your thoughts to the points made after the presentation of results in the critical analysis section.

Description of sample

Fifty clinical/fieldwork educators completed and returned the questionnaire (75% return rate). Twenty-one respondents were occupational therapists and 29 were physiotherapists. Fifteen occupational therapists had up to five years' supervising experience compared to 21 physiotherapists. Nine occupational therapists had over five years' supervising experience compared to six physiotherapists. Both occupational therapy and physiotherapy clinical/fieldwork educators have had a wide range of experience in working with students. A factor that both occupational therapists and physiotherapists have in common is that the majority supervise students single-handed. Occupational therapists tend to supervise students at all stages of training, while the physiotherapists tend to offer placements for students at one stage of training.

The results from the questionnaire will be presented in order to

Table 17.1 Summary of ratings for briefing exercise and assessment form

How useful:	Range	Mode	Mean	How easy:	Range	Mode	Mean
Description of course (OT)	4–10	8	7.6	Using assessment form (OT)	5–10	7	7.6
Description of course (PT)	5–10	8	7.7	Using assessment form (PT)	5–9	8	7.3
Grading exercise (OT)	4–10	8 and 10	7.2	Grading exercise (OT)	3–10	8	7.2
Grading exercise (PT)	4–10	8	8.2	Grading exercise (PT)	3–8	8	7

ascertain general feedback from clinical/fieldwork educators regarding the perceived value and effectiveness of the briefing session, and particularly the use of the case studies. Information that could be used to improve either the briefing session or the assessment form will also be highlighted.

Experience of briefing sessions

The information in Table 17.1 reveals that, overall, both occupational therapists and physiotherapists appear to have found the briefing session useful, particularly the grading exercise. The range indicates, however, that some respondents did not find the experience very useful, with ratings as low as 4. Similar results are achieved for the ratings of how easy the assessment form and grading exercise were. The large ranges, particularly for the ratings of the grading exercise, indicate a wide variation in responses. Some therapists found the exercise very easy while others found it very hard.

An analysis of what respondents felt they had learnt from the briefing session revealed four common factors that were listed by occupational therapists and physiotherapists:

1. *Grading and assessment issues:* learning how to use the assessment form, criteria for grading the student and the need for reliability.
2. *Expectations of the School:* understanding the School and student's expectations of the placement and the clinical/fieldwork educator.
3. *Content and nature of student learning:* getting information about the course, what level the student is at and the relationship between occupational therapy and physiotherapy students at Southshore.
4. *Agreement with peers:* having a discussion with other clinical/fieldwork educators that helped to focus on potential areas of difficulty, reassurance that they had graded the case studies very similarly to other clinicians.

The occupational therapists raised the two additional issues of:

1. *Refreshment of skills:* the briefing session was a useful revision exercise.

Table 17.2   Summary of ratings for how easy therapists found it to grade students

How easy:	Range	Mode	Mean	How prepared:	Range	Mode	Mean
Grading student (OT)	4–9	7 and 8	6.7	Prepared for marking real student (OT)	5–9	7	7.2
Grading student (PT)	3–9	7	6.8	Prepared for marking real student (PT)	3–10	7	6.8
Using assessment form (OT)	4–10	7	7.3				
Using assessment form (PT)	4–9	8	6.6				

2. *Problem students:* gaining new ideas for dealing with problems early.

The physiotherapists raised one additional issue of:

1. *Information about the School:* understanding the general running and administration of the School, including the structure of the course.

Analysis of the most common critical factors for the clinical/fieldwork educators when grading the hypothetical case studies related to the process and experience of grading (objectivity and reliability, criteria and hypothetical versus real) moreso than qualities of the student.

Grading students on placement

From the data in Table 17.2 it is observed that both occupational therapists and physiotherapists found it reasonably easy to grade students on placement, using the assessment form. Both groups, however, found it slightly less easy to grade a real student compared with a hypothetical one. For example, occupational therapists gave an average of 6.7 for grading a real students, compared with 7.2 for a hypothetical one. While the averages for how prepared clinical/fieldwork educators felt the briefing sessions made them are reassuringly quite high, it is concerning that the range was quite high, particularly for the physiotherapists. This suggests a wide variation in opinions concerning preparedness.

Personal comments

An analysis of the comments made by respondents at the end of the questionnaire reflects the findings of the pilot studies and briefing sessions. For example, some comments reflect the differences in grading for A students and Fail students:

'Grading a student is much easier when they are excellent but it is much harder when they are D level or Fail'.

Other comments related to issues such as:

• Working in a group during the assessment exercise.

'Very helpful in standardizing grading'.
'Good to see the consistency of grading between educators'.
'It has been useful to ensure that one separates clinical/fieldwork competence from effort put in by the student'.

• Reality of grading a hypothetical case study.

'Found hypothetical grading very difficult, you would continually assess student over the weeks and relate their interaction to others to grade'.
'Obviously not the same as grading a student face to face'.

• The design of the assessment form.

'I did not find the form that helpful, there were areas that were not relevant at particular periods of training'.
'Did not like the term adequate, to me this means that only the minimum necessary has been achieved'.

• Importance of reliability.

'Briefing sessions were very fair in helping standardize the marking'.
'Grading students is an enormous responsibility'.

Critical analysis of the sample results section

Readers will remember that the sample results section was not perfect. Hence there are plenty of comments to make in critically reviewing it. The start of the results section cues us in well as to how the results are going to be used and the context in which they were collected. For example, we can note the 75% return rate for questionnaires – this is pretty good.

This sample results section also does a good job at summarizing and focusing. With the tables we are told what the main points are and with the open responses the main factors and themes are identified for us.

There has been some attempt to interpret or respond to the results. For example, indicating that the personal comments reflected the findings of the briefing sessions. However, the author has on occasion mixed interpretation with subjectivity: 'While the averages for how prepared clinical/fieldwork educators felt the briefing sessions made them are *reassuringly* quite high, it is *concerning* that the range was quite high'.

There are also some problems with the way the data have been presented. For example, while the tables present figures for the mean and mode, the mode is not referred to in the interpretation of the tables. It is therefore not clear why they are presented in addition to the means. Tables 17.1 and 17.2 are also four tables merged into two. This needs to be made clearer with a line or break down the middle of the tables. In presenting the themes that emerged from the personal comments the author has chosen to give a couple of example quotes. While this may be illustrative, we perhaps need some indication of how representative these quotes are of the whole data set.

The final point to note is that the results section ended quite abruptly. It would have been helpful for the author to have reminded the reader what the research question was and highlighted the main findings in order to indicate whether the research question has been answered.

Key points

1. Writing up your results may be a difficult process if you do not readdress the purpose of the study or if the results cause us to question the quality of the study.
2. Writing up your results can be a very creative process if you are able to gain 'control' of the data.
3. There are seven main sections of a standard research report: title, abstract, introduction, method, results, discussion and conclusion, references and appendices.
4. The format and style of your research report will differ depending on your target audience.

References

Brodie, D.A., Williams, J.G. and Glynn Owens, R. (1994). *Research Methods for the Health Sciences*. Harwood Academic Publishers.

Currier, D.P. (1990). *Elements of Research in Physiotherapy*, 3rd Edn. Williams and Wilkins.

Drummond, A. (1996). *Research Methods for Therapists*. Chapman & Hall.

French, S. (1993). *Practical Research: A Guide for Therapists*. Butterworth-Heinemann.

Maykut, P. and Morehouse, R. (1996). *Beginning Qualitative Research: A Philosophic and Practical Guide*. The Falmer Press.

Seale, J., Gallagher, C. and Grisbrooke, J. (1996). Fieldwork educator training: design and evaluation of an educational package. *British Journal of Occupational Therapy*, **59**, 529–534.

Strauss, A.L. (1995). *Qualitative Analysis for Social Scientists*. Cambridge University Press.

Complementary reading

Ballinger, C., Curtin, M., Eakin, P., Hollis,V., Nicol, M. and Telford, R. (1996). Writing an abstract. *British Journal of Occupational Therapy*, **59**, 33–35.

Bell, J. (1987). *Doing Your Research Project*. Open University Press.

Parry, A. (1993). How to construct an outline for a research report. *Physiotherapy*, **79**, 257–258.

18 Writing up your research: discussing your results

The purpose of a discussion section

In Chapter 17 we noted that the purpose of a discussion section in an article or report is to interpret and debate your findings. A discussion section usually starts off with a brief reiteration of what your main research findings were. You may then move on to state how your results fit in with the findings from other related research. This may involve mentioning studies that either corroborate or contradict your results. In addition to comparing your results with those of other researchers you may need to place the results in a theoretical context. Your results may clarify or extend an existing body of knowledge or you may feel that you wish to produce a new theoretical framework in which to place your results.

Towards the end of a discussion section you may need to consider any problems with the project which may influence the interpretation of the findings. For example, if your results are not what you expected or contradict other results then you may need to find an explanation for the discrepancy. This will usually involve considering problems with your methodology but may also require you to question your assumptions, research questions or hypotheses.

The final part of a discussion section involves identifying implications for future research. This may involve indicating the possible follow-up studies that may be carried out to build on your findings and clarify them further, or it may involve redesigning the original study in order to do a better job and perhaps get clearer results. The key to writing a successful discussion section is keeping the discussion focused on your research question and not going beyond the scope of your findings and making giant leaps or claims that your project cannot support.

Drummond (1996) notes that the discussion may be considered or visualized as an inverted funnel shape. The first part or wedge involves interpreting the results of the study. The second larger wedge involves relating the project to other work in the area, and the final largest wedge involves discussing the general application and relevance of the findings.

Explaining results and admitting problems

Many of us treat the writing up stage as some kind of public relations exercise where we have to convince readers and colleagues that our research project was flawless and perfect. In one sense that is very understandable; none of us wants to admit that our project was useless and a total waste of time. But, on the other hand, this is the real world and there is no such thing as a perfect, flawless research project. Things go wrong for even the most experienced professional researcher. What makes a good researcher is the ability to recognize when and how their results may have been influenced by unexpected factors. If we hear a market salesman trying to sell 'genuine' Rolex watches for £5, most of would hear the alarm bells ringing and assume that they must have fallen off the back of a lorry and probably won't work for very long. Equally, if we hear a researcher claiming that their research project had no problems whatsoever, then we should hear the alarm bells ringing and approach their results with caution.

If you are writing up your research as part of a student project or dissertation then the problems that you may need to report are varied. They might include participants withdrawing, the research sample not being large enough to make generalizations, poor quality questionnaires, bad timing of data collection or having a project that is simply over-ambitious. But as French (1993) quite rightly says, beware of overdoing your reports of problems and misfortunes. She warns that you may make yourself look like a victim or someone with an axe to grind. Either of these two scenarios may give the impression that you are trying to avoid taking responsibility for the project. With student projects the marker will probably be looking for evidence that you have reflected on the experience of conducting the project and have learnt something from doing it which you can apply to the next project you conduct. Identifying problems with your project is not about apportioning or admitting blame but asking yourself 'If I was to do this project again, what would I do differently?'.

If you are writing your results up in order to publish in a journal or present at a conference then you will still need to consider problems with your study. As this consideration is happening in a more public arena then the way in which you address the potential problems with your study may be more measured and framed in a slightly different language.

In the rest of this chapter a sample discussion section will be presented. A critique of the discussion will then be offered in order to highlight the issues raised in the introduction.

A sample discussion section

The sample discussion section is interpreting the sample results that were presented in Chapter 17. The discussion is based on the work conducted by Seale, Gallagher and Grisbrooke (1996). Just as the sample results section was not perfect, neither is this sample discussion section. When you are reading the sample discussion section ask yourself the following questions:

- Does it include a brief reiteration of the results?
- Does it state how the results fit in with other findings?
- Does it clarify an existing body of knowledge?
- Does it consider methodological problems?
- Does it identify future research work?

Readers please note that for the purposes of brevity only question-naire results were presented in Chapter 17; however, in the discussion section results from a grading exercise and interviews will be referred to as well. The discussion section will also refer to tables that you will not have seen. To recap, the study in question was designed to investigate the usefulness of an educational package for training clinical fieldwork educators. The educational package consisted of case studies of hypothetical students on clinical placement. The pro-ducers of the package were keen to investigate whether the case studies were a useful educational tool in helping clinical/fieldwork educators familiarize themselves with the clinical/fieldwork assess-ment criteria.

Discussion

The purpose of the study was to develop and evaluate an educational package that could be used in the briefing sessions. The results of the grading exercise in the briefing session will be used to evaluate the usefulness of the case studies. The results of the questionnaires and interviews will be used to evaluate the briefing sessions and the assessment form and consider possible changes to both which may be required. Possibilities for future investigations will be considered along with the feasibility of applying the same model of clinical/fieldwork organization to other professional degree courses including those outside of the health sciences.

Grading hypothetical cases

Analysis of the data from briefing sessions B, C and D reveals quite high levels of agreement with the expected grades, with mean levels of agreement ranging from 56.8% to 98%. Respondents to both the questionnaire and interview commented upon this relatively high level of agreement. The clinicians who commented felt that it was re-assuring to see that a large number of them were giving the same grades to the case studies. This appears to reflect a real concern, particularly from the new clinical/fieldwork educators that the clinicians should be reliable and consistent markers.

There were, however, fluctuations in gradings for certain case studies or sections of the case studies. For example, the figures in Tables 7 and 8 reveal grade ranges as high as five (A–E) and mean percentage agreement as low as 15%. A small number of clinicians, notably the more experienced ones, seem to pick up on inconsistencies in grading during the briefing session. It may be these inconsistencies that they were noticing.

Attempts to explain such fluctuations might focus on the relative supervisory experience of the clinicians who attended the briefing sessions. In total, for all three briefing sessions, there were 75 clinicians who had no experience of working with students, 116 who had up to five years' experience and 69 clinicians who had over five years' experience. These figures indicate that inexperienced clinical/fieldwork educators do not outnumber experienced clinical/fieldwork educators. A closer analysis of the figures, notably Table 6, reveals very little differences in the mean percentage of agreement between the three groups of clinicians, despite the fact that inexperienced clinicians outnumbered the very experienced clinicians (27 to 16).

While the briefing sessions were being conducted it was noted that a lot of physiotherapists who had not supervised a student before were attending. For example, for briefing session D the percentage of inexperienced PTs in the group was 35% compared with 14% for OTs, while the percentage of experienced PTs was 5% compared with 45% for OTs. However, the difference between OTs and PTs in mean percentage agreement was not great (76.9% compared with 71.4%).

It would seem that the fluctuations in grading couldn't be easily attributed to the supervisory experience of the clinicians *per se*. It may not be important whether or not the clinicians have supervised students before; what may be important is their experience of using the School's particular assessment form. It is different to other assessment forms that the clinicians may have come across. This issue will be addressed further when the assessment form is evaluated more fully later.

While there were generally high levels of agreement in the briefing session, patterns of grading were observed which would need addressing in further briefing sessions. For example, it was very encouraging that the clinicians were able to recognize very readily an A grade student and a Fail student. However, when clinicians are assessing real students, there have been occasions when clinical/fieldwork educators have required a lot of support in order to fail a student and, conversely, where they have been very reluctant to give an A. The difficulty clinicians have in failing students may reflect an anxiety that they do not want to be responsible for the student failing his or her degree. This is a responsibility which they feel they have had placed on them now that grades from clinical/fieldwork placements contribute to the classification of the degree. Clinicians' anxiety about their ability to fail students was noted by Cross (1992) in a survey of clinical/fieldwork educators' learning needs. A common question raised by clinicians was 'Do all clinicians fail students when they think they should?'. As most clinicians wish to see clinical/fieldwork contribute to the degree, this is an issue that must be resolved.

Some clinicians made comment about the difficulty of grading low-achieving students and inspection of those comments may help us to understand why clinicians in all the case studies found it harder to grade the D grade case study and, therefore, why agreement levels were relatively so low.

> 'Grading a student is much easier when they are excellent; it is much harder when they are at a D or Fail level'.

Comments from the clinicians also reveal a potential difference in the grading patterns of clinicians for real and hypothetical A grade students. When talking about the case studies, one clinician in the interview said:

'The ones that were really excellent, I thought, I've never had a student like that'.

Students are coming back from placement reporting that their clinical/ fieldwork educator had said that they never give students A grades. This is despite the plain statement made during all clinical briefing sessions that the School expects it to be possible for a good student to be awarded an A grade. For some clinicians there appears to be a belief that in order to get an A you have to be functioning at a Junior or Basic Grade level, in other words as if you were already qualified. Yet the assessment forms were designed to reflect performance at different stages of student development, so that it is possible to get an A. While clinicians seem very able to recognize what theoretically should be an A grade student, they do not always seem to operate in this way when working with real students. Burrows (1989) suggests that it is easier to identify when someone is incompetent and has fallen below a certain standard than it is to recognize when someone is competent and achieving a certain standard.

Clinicians also seemed to struggle with case studies where the grades for the individual skill sections were not the same as the overall grade (the B grade case study in the briefing session, for example). This difficulty may reflect the fact that some clinicians may be used to the assessment forms from other schools, where they are only required to give an overall grade.

The briefing session

Results from the questionnaire reveal good ratings for the briefing sessions (see Table 11). The clinicians liked the fact that the briefing session enabled them to learn about the assessment form, the expectations of the School, student progress and knowledge and how their peers assess clinical performance. This positive evaluation is also identified in the interview data. The format and presentation was well received and considered to be timely, informative and relevant in content. The grading exercise was seen to form the core of the session and had an impact, particularly for the new clinical/fieldwork educators. For new clinical/fieldwork educators the opportunity to use the assessment form was a positive preparation for taking students. Finding that their grading of a student coincided with that of other clinical/fieldwork educators had a powerful and positive impact.

While overall positive feedback about the briefing session was obtained there are areas of concern. The wide range of ratings noted in the questionnaire data (Tables 11 and 12) suggests that the briefing session is not meeting everyone's needs. Information from the interviews may present an explanation for this. In the interview a number of experienced clinical/fieldwork educators said that they did not learn anything that they did not know already, although some did accept that it was a useful revision exercise. While experienced clinical/fieldwork educators may believe that the briefing session was less useful, we have already noted that their levels of agreement were not significantly higher than those of inexperienced clinicians. This suggests that the School may need to 'sell' the briefing session rather better to the experienced clinicians and persuade them that they can learn something new from it, particularly as an introduction to the School is included in the briefing session. Experienced clinical/fieldwork educators may not be new to working with students but they are new to the School and its clinical/fieldwork system. From a discussion of the results it would appear that future briefing sessions would need to:

1. Address positive and negative concerns about uniformity and reliability in marking – within the briefing sessions and on placement.
2. Address the issue of grading a real student and a hypothetical student – and give clinicians permission and support to give students As and Fails.
3. Address the issue of giving different grades in each section of the form and how this may differ from other assessment forms.
4. Attempt to address everyone's needs, irrespective of experience. It may be possible to 'brief' experienced and inexperienced clinicians separately, although this has disadvantages as well as advantages.
5. Be an optimum size to facilitate discussion and shared experiences.

Some of these issues can also be addressed in the study days and educational workshops that are run by the School. A follow-up session after working with students may also be useful so that clinical/fieldwork educators can discuss assessment issues in the light of working with a real student. Staff who run briefing sessions will also need to be trained to cope with the broad discussions that may arise from giving As and Fails to students. It may be advantageous to involve experienced clinical/fieldwork educators in the running of the briefing sessions.

Assessment form

From the questionnaire data there was evidence from both professions that the assessment form was reasonably easy to use (see Table 11). From the interview data there was evidence that, on the whole, the assessment form was considered to be comprehensive in coverage. Giving clinicians the opportunity to write comments as well as give a grade also extended the flexibility of the assessment form for the clinicians. The occupational therapists were, on the whole, happy with the grades elicited by the form. Where there was criticism, it was when a student could be given a higher grade than was actually merited using the form. Some physiotherapists, on the other hand, felt that the form had not allowed them to offer sufficiently high grades. The implication of this is that the physiotherapists have a tendency to mark higher than occupational therapists. This is not an issue which had emerged during the briefing sessions but it may need to be addressed. An inspection of the grades given to real students on placement reveals that the physiotherapy grades do not follow as normal a distribution as the occupational therapy ones and are slightly skewed towards the upper grades of A and B.

Clinicians made very few specific recommendations for changing the form; however, a very common problem that was noted in the interview and the questionnaire was a dissatisfaction with the use of just three standards to grade each performance criteria on the assessment form (weak, adequate, excellent). Clinicians seemed particularly unhappy with the definition of adequate and how it was used to distinguish between different grades. Changing these standards may help clinicians to distinguish between D and Fail, and indeed may help clinicians give As more often.

Overall the clinicians made little issue over the division of the form into four skill areas, with just one interviewee talking about changing the weighting of the interpersonal and management sections. It would be interesting to explore further reasons why clinicians were in strong agreement with the expected grades for safety and management and less so for interpersonal and clinical skills. Ellis (1993) proposes that 'competence must refer to the total of observable behaviours that occur in professional practice, categorized and specified in relation to measurable standards'. There are, nevertheless, 'unobservable attributes, capacities, dispositions, attitudes and values' that are frequently submerged and unobservable which influence a student's behaviour and clinical performance. Perhaps interpersonal and clinical skills are skills that fall into this category. This would certainly seem worthy of further investigation.

From a discussion of the results it would appear that specific issues to consider in reviewing the assessment form would be:

1. The widening of the three standards used to assess performance criteria.
2. The behaviours being assessed in each of the four sections and the desirability of including different weighting.
3. Methods of making the distinction between the grade bands clearer, such as making the percentages attributed to each grade explicit.

Replication of the educational package

Occupational therapy and physiotherapy degree courses are not alone in incorporating a clinical/fieldwork component. Medicine, nursing and social work degree courses, to name but a few, are courses that require students to demonstrate clinical/fieldwork competence. This competence is frequently assessed by clinicians other than lecturing staff. Other health professions such as medical and nursing staff have engaged in a debate regarding effective clinical/fieldwork educator behaviours (Stritter *et al.*, 1975; Wong and Wong, 1980; Wolf and Turner, 1989). The debate has also focused on methods of achieving reliable assessment of student performance. In considering whether other degree courses could replicate the educational package evaluated in this study, three key points need to be taken into consideration:

1. The hypothetical case studies will need to reflect whatever assessment form/system is being used by the professional group in question.
2. The educational establishment will need a firm commitment to a collaborative and ongoing training programme for clinical/fieldwork educators (Cross, 1994), including a shared and negotiated assessment form which will be reviewed and evaluated on a regular basis (Swinehart and Meyers, 1993) and the close involvement of clinical tutors.
3. The suggested changes to the briefing sessions and the assessment form highlighted in this study will need to be noted and incorporated where it is considered appropriate.

Future action/research

Analysis and discussion of the results of this study reveal several tasks that will need to be undertaken in order to disseminate information and build on the work already completed. Results of the study can be fed back to clinical/fieldwork educators by giving presentations at study days and to clinical/fieldwork organising groups, and providing copies of this report (or a summary) to key personnel such as clinical/fieldwork co-ordinators within local health care organizations.

The implications of the study for related professional courses could be fed back by inviting key personnel to a presentation/seminar and providing copies of this report (or a summary) to key personnel such as clinical/fieldwork co-ordinators within other educational departments.

Results from this study have highlighted further research and investigations that are required in order to gain greater insight into the training needs of clinical/fieldwork educators. Possible steps include:

1. Replicate the studies presented, incorporating the recommended changes, and evaluate the success and effectiveness of the changes.
2. Address validity issues in grading clinical/fieldwork experiences. This study has addressed to some extent the reliability of clinical/fieldwork assessment and it would now seem appropriate to examine issues of validity. Is the assessment form measuring what it is supposed to be measuring? Are we all working to the same definitions of A, B, C, D and Fail? This analysis can be achieved by examining data collected on section 3 of the questionnaire.
3. In order to identify useful topics for future training courses it would be advantageous to investigate in more detail the 'grading' behaviour of clinical/fieldwork educators and factors that influence their grading of students, such as half-time and full-time grading. This analysis can be achieved by examining data collected on sections 3 and 4 of the questionnaire and 2 and 3 of the interview.

The use of hypothetical case studies within a training programme for clinical/fieldwork educators has proved to be a useful exercise and has provided a valuable insight into how and why clinical/fieldwork educators award the grades they do to students. While the results from this study have elicited, on the whole, positive comments about the briefing sessions and the assessment form, there are areas which require improvement and further work. The School and the research team are committed to investigating the areas identified more fully in future research and development projects.

Critical analysis of the sample discussion section

The sample discussion section handled a lot of data quite well. Rather than summarize all the results at the beginning of the discussion, pertinent results were referred to throughout the discussion. The discussion of the results was well structured. The reader was cued in to focus on three main areas, the grading of the case studies, the briefing session and the assessment form. What you will not have been able to do in reading the discussion section is to refer back to the results section in order to ascertain whether the author's interpretations and claims are justified by the data. It is worth checking any discussion section you read in order to see if objectivity is being compromised by personal opinion. We very often accept discussions in research reports, particularly ones published in journals, as offering credible and legitimate explanations for obtained results. French (1993) reminds us of the phenomenon she calls the 'power of the printed word', whereby the results of published studies and the interpretations put upon them can be accepted uncritically and therefore greatly influence our thinking.

The discussion also does a good job of trying to explain some of the results and highlighting points that require future work and consideration. For example, it attempts to explore why clinicians were strongly in agreement with the expected grades for safety and management but less so for interpersonal and clinical skills. However, the discussion does not attempt to identify any limitations of the study such as generalizability to other OT or PT courses or the representativeness of the sample. This may be a bit concerning.

The discussion makes some attempt to place the results in a theoretical context by making a few references back to other literature, although you may feel that this is possibly a bit limited. A closer inspection will reveal that the literature being referred to was not that of previous studies, whereby the results of one study could be compared with another. Rather, the literature was more like that of opinion or discussion papers. So, for example, in discussing reasons why less agreement was obtained for interpersonal and clinical skills than for safety and management the work of Ellis in 1993 is referred to. This work is a book called *Professional Competence and Quality Assurance in the Caring Professions*. In this book Ellis uses other literature to build a theory or model of what exactly clinical competence is. Given the relative lack of published therapy research projects it is likely that only a minority of discussion sections will be able to include a lengthy debate about which therapy studies confirm or reject current findings. What we must try and avoid, however, is the temptation to use lack of therapy research as an excuse for not placing our interpretations into some kind of context. If we are unable to compare our results with other results then we can compare them against published ideas, views and arguments, as this discussion has done.

If we apply all the criteria laid down in the introduction to this chapter then this discussion is not a 'perfect discussion'. What it does well is attempt to explain the results. What it fails to do is identify any problems or issues with the methodologies of the study.

Key points

1. The purpose of a discussion section is to interpret and debate your findings.
2. A discussion section should include a brief reiteration of results, state how results fit with other findings, clarify an existing body of knowledge, consider methodological problems and identify future research work.
3. In attempting to explain our results we should not be afraid of admitting problems with the research.
4. Try not to use a lack of therapy research as an excuse for not placing your results in a theoretical context.

References

Drummond, A. (1996). *Research Methods for Therapists.* Chapman & Hall.

French, S. (1993). Telling. In *Reflecting on Research Practice.* (P. Shakespeare, D. Atkinson and S. French, eds), pp. 119–130. Open University Press.

Seale, J., Gallagher, C. and Grisbrooke, J. (1996). Fieldwork educator training: design and evaluation of an educational package. *British Journal of Occupational Therapy*, **59**, 529–534.

Complementary reading

Hicks, C. (1995). *Research for Physiotherapists. Project Design and Analysis.* Churchill Livingstone. Chapter 11: Writing up the research for publication.

19 Disseminating research findings

The need for dissemination

Dissemination generally means to spread ideas widely. In the research field, dissemination means to inform a targeted audience about the results of your research. It has often been stated that dissemination is a neglected part of the research process (French, 1993a). Dissemination of research results is seen as important for a variety of reasons: so therapy can grow and develop, to contribute to the body of knowledge, so our ideas are critically analysed by other people and to contribute to the reduction of the gap between theory and practice (Dickson, 1994). If the results of research are not disseminated then the researcher may be considered 'derelict in his responsibilities' (Currier, 1990, p. 290) and essentially will have wasted a lot of time and energy if no one is to know the outcome of his work. It is generally accepted that if results are not disseminated they are of little value.

There may be many reasons why researchers fail to disseminate their work. Currier (1990) identified a fear of rejection, along with the additional time and energy required for writing studies up, while Cormack (1994, p. 132) highlights a frequent phenomenon in therapy research, that of assuming someone else will do it if you don't. Writing is often perceived as 'something which an unspecified "they" do, and which is beyond the scope of most professionals'.

If you are able to choose a dissemination method that you feel comfortable with then perhaps you will feel less anxious. If you are able to understand the context in which reviewers make comments on your work, then again you may be less afraid to submit your work for peer review and scrutiny. There are probably few solutions to the problem of not having the time and energy to write up your research; we don't have the power to put the clocks back or turn you into 'wonderperson'! However, if you are able to target your audience effectively then you may reduce the chances of your efforts being a waste of time. This chapter will highlight the different methods of dissemination that a health care professional may use, discuss ways of targeting your audience and consider how to deal with feedback or criticism of your work.

Different methods of dissemination

There is a wide variety of ways of disseminating the results of your study. During the research study you may arrange regular talks, seminars, newsletters or progress reports. After the research study has finished you may wish to try and inform or change practice by producing training packs and booklets, taking part in radio and TV interviews or holding meetings with relevant pressure groups. In a more academic environment writing is perhaps the most common method used for disseminating the results of research. In addition there are alternative methods that may complement or substitute a written report, such as the conference abstract, talks and presentations, posters and publications in the popular press.

The journal article

The format of a journal article will be similar to the standard research report layout outlined in Chapter 17, though the length is likely to be condensed due to specified limits on the number of words. Check the appropriate journal's guide for contributors for details of acceptable style and structure and length of articles. It is advisable to write with a particular journal in mind, so have a good look at the journal and see if your work is appropriate and 'fits'. If the article is highly specialized, it will be necessary to choose journals that either deal with that speciality or have a broad readership (Cormack, 1994).

Conference abstract

A conference abstract is a brief summary of the research project, which is submitted to conference organizers (see Figure, 19.1 for example). The abstract will often be peer reviewed to decide whether to invite

The School of Occupational Therapy and Physiotherapy (SOTP) at the University of Southampton has an innovative assessment programme which aims to produce professionals who can perform as clinicians, educators, managers and researchers. The assessments vary in nature from traditional written examinations to oral presentations; examples include the Objective Structured Practical Examination and the Structured Evaluation of a Self-Directed Learning Experience (Triple Jump). This assessment programme is considered to promote a balance in skills and knowledge and avoids disadvantaging students who perform poorly in one particular type of assessment. This is critical considering the wide range of applicants that SOTP attracts. Applicants vary in their age, experience and academic qualifications. Whatever their backgrounds, when students join SOTP they are usually highly committed to becoming practising clinicians. This commitment appears to translate to a strong motivation to pass assessments. Reflections from the presenters over the four years that the programme has been running has lead to a questioning of whether this motivation to pass is at the expense of a motivation to learn. The aims of the session will be to describe the assessment programme at the School, to identify possible influences of such an assessment programme on student motivation, to present the results from a survey investigating the reflections and opinions of third year students on their varied assessment programme and to discuss the nature of the motivation elicited by the different assessment methods.

Figure 19.1 Example of a conference abstract (Chapman, Davey and Seale, 1997). (See also Ballinger *et al.*, 1996 for an example of a conference abstract published in a journal.)

the writer to give a full oral presentation based on the content of the abstract. The abstract may also be published in the conference proceedings or a related journal. Currier (1990) notes that calls for conference abstracts are often put out months before you have completed the research that you want to report on. For this reason he warns readers of conference abstracts to be wary of published abstracts which may be based on incomplete studies.

Talks and presentations

You may choose a talk or a presentation as a method of dissemination if you wish to present your work at a conference where the audience is fellow practitioners or researchers. Equally, you may choose a talk or presentation if you wish to present your findings in a meeting of stakeholders or people for whom the results are pertinent.

While the audience in a meeting of stakeholders may have an interest or stake in your study, they may not be totally familiar with your research methodology or the jargon that accompanies research. Such presentations will therefore need to take into account a lack of knowledge on the part of the audience. For example, Maykut and Morehouse (1996) report how they used slides taken throughout the course of a project to illustrate the research process to audiences who were unfamiliar with qualitative research.

In a meeting that you have called to present your findings to stakeholders or interested parties there is likely to be less formal protocol involved than for a presentation given at a conference. At conferences you often have time limits, an appointed chairperson, recommendations for how many slides to show and so on.

The skill of presenting research findings orally is to make the talk interesting, stimulating and coherent (French, 1993a). The key to achieving this centres on how you use your notes and audio-visual aids. It is often inadvisable to read directly from your notes, word for word, as this tends to sound quite boring to the listener and may serve to 'switch them off'. Rather than reading verbatim from your notes you may find it useful to use cue cards on which you just write down the main points that you need to remember and then use them as a cue to expand further in your talk. Using a variety of audio-visual aids may help you to hold the attention of the audience. However, if you are going to use a range of aids then allow plenty of time to familiarize yourself with the room and the equipment. If you are fumbling around with black-out equipment and pointers then you will quickly lose the attention of the audience. Whatever kind of aid you are using (slides, overhead projector, video, etc.) you need to make sure there is an accurate match between what is on your aids and what you are saying. There is often a temptation to overfill slides, particularly with large tables. Resist this temptation and keep the slides relatively uncluttered, using large bulleted points and highly summarized information. You can always expand on the information presented in a slide during your talk.

Conference talks often have a time limit so you need to be very selective in what you choose to present. The most common mistake is to cram too much in. Brodie *et al.* (1994) note that a common fault in less experienced presenters is to spend too much time on methodology to the detriment of the results. They suggest that you assume your audience wants results and argue that you should be prepared to spend as much time as is necessary to disseminate the results clearly. The main message is to concentrate on major themes rather than detail. If you need to provide extensive detail you can perhaps provide a hand-out at the end of the talk, or refer the audience to your more detailed article in the conference proceedings.

Another aspect of talks and presentations is dealing with questions from the audience. Question time is often built into formal conference presentations. For less formal presentations and meetings you may like to encourage the audience to express their own views and ask questions. Throwing the floor open to questions and criticism can provide useful feedback which you can use to inform your own practice in the future and highlights the point that dissemination is not a one-way process where you give and others receive. Inviting questions takes courage because there is always a fear that you will not be able to answer the questions and that you will therefore look foolish.

Poster

A poster is often a popular way of displaying research findings at conferences. It enables people to look at the research in their own time and talk to researchers on a one-to-one basis. In a conference poster just the essential points are displayed as space is at a premium. A poster is likely to include the title, purpose, brief methods, major results and conclusions.

The size of the poster and details of presentation (size of lettering, area, etc.) are usually stipulated by the conference organizers. In order to grab a conference delegate's attention as he or she is walking around the exhibition area your poster needs to be striking and easy to read. This is often easy to achieve through the use of desk-top publishing or presentation software.

Popular press

The popular press in research terms includes newspapers and newsletters that would be considered 'lightweight'. Articles are often not peer reviewed; instead the editor will normally decide whether to publish your work. A report in a popular newspaper may not need to be so formally structured as a journal article but is still likely to have a set word limit and a style template. Check any instructions for authors that are given in the newspaper or contact the editor. Because more people are likely to read popular newspapers than academic journals this method of dissemination may be more satisfying for you (French, 1993a). French warns us, however, that publishing in the popular press runs the risk of possible distortion (sensationalized headlines, crude editing, etc.) and a lack of recognition in academic circles.

Table 19.1 Choosing a dissemination method to match your audience

Audience	Type of dissemination
Examiners/ commissioners/funders/ ethics committee	Dissertation, executive summary, short report, presentation (viva, informal or conference).
Participants	Letters, presentation at open meeting.
Colleagues	Presentation or seminar to department/branch/ special interest group, article in newsletter, national conference paper or poster, paper in professional journal.
Wider professional audience	Conference paper or poster, paper in professional or academic journal, research review in a newsletter or 'medical comic'.
Wider public audience	Paper in popular press, TV/radio interview, training packs, booklets.

Targeting your audience

Table 19.1 briefly summarizes the different types of dissemination you might use depending on the audience you wish to target. It is unlikely that you are going to rely on one method of dissemination alone. You are likely to choose a combination of methods. Undergraduate students, for example, usually have to produce a dissertation, but there is an increasing trend towards encouraging students to present their findings at a conference or to publish their study in a professional journal.

Being peer reviewed

The use of a peer review system for evaluating what is being disseminated is increasing. We are used to journal articles being peer reviewed, but other publications that may also be peer reviewed include conference abstracts and project reports for funded research. Journal articles and conference abstracts are reviewed in order to decide whether the author's work is worthy of a wider audience. Project reports from funded research are peer reviewed in order to decide the quality of the research (methodology, originality, problems, etc.), the value of the research (practical implications, value for money, etc.) and the impact of the research (general, economic or health benefits for example). While you get feedback from reviewers who have considered your journal article or conference abstract, you may not get feedback from reviewers who have considered your project report.

The majority of the literature focuses on the peer review system for journal articles. In this system there are three main players: the reviewer, the editor and the author. The role of the reviewer is to decide whether the article is worthy of publication and whether principles of good writing have been followed. Reviewers check for accuracy, interest and contribution to therapy (Currier, 1990). It is perhaps useful to note that reviewers are unpaid and give up their valuable time to read manuscripts. The role of the editor will vary from journal to journal but, on the whole, their job is to educate and guide the author without discouraging them (Currier, 1990). The role of the author is to take on board any comments made by the reviewers and make appropriate changes.

Reviewers will offer comments and suggestions in varying amounts of detail and, since the comments are often made anonymously, there can be a tendency towards curtness (see Figure 19.2 for an example). However, the feedback that an author receives will range from straightforward acceptance without modifications, acceptance with modifications or rejection.

A rejection does not necessarily mean that the work is awful; it may not be relevant for the journal in question (Brodie *et al.*, 1994). Cormack (1994, p. 143) offers some advice for those authors who experience rejection at the hands of reviewers and editors:

> 'In the event of an editor rejecting a manuscript which has been submitted for the first time, the temptation to throw it away or to write an angry letter to the editor must be resisted . . . Rejection slips are not the end of the road for a particular manuscript. Their contents should be studied carefully and learned from'.

If a paper has been accepted subject to minor revision the editor might not show the revised paper to the reviewers. If the paper has required major revisions then the reviewers are likely to be invited to offer comment on those revisions. Brodie *et al.* (1994) advise that, when responding to specific referees' comments, it is essential to

---

An interesting paper that would benefit from a clearer focus and editing. The content, however, seems too ambitious. Also, the headings suggest a scientific, rather than descriptive, article. If so, more attention needs to be paid to research details and terminology.

The abstract is too long with duplication, lack of variety in the language and changes in tense.

Is all the background information necessary in the introduction? Is it pertinent to the focus or really a comprehensive review of the literature?

The methodology section requires more detail, justification, research terminology and structure if retained as part of a scientific paper. For example, selection of sample and format of questionnaire, e.g. ranking or Likert scales.

The tables in the results section were unclear due to omission of details about the scales used or number of respondents. The final paragraph in this section contains a more precise, concise style which could be extended to the whole paper.

The discussion needs a more scholarly style. The conclusions are abrupt and context specific.

The paper is addressing a really important topic.

Figure 19.2   Hypothetical example of a reviewer's comments.

cross-reference each comment with your response and outline in a letter to the editor the changes you have made.

With three players in the arena there is scope for disagreement, particularly on the part of the author. The author may not be able to accept the criticisms or may find it impossible to undertake the recommendations given. Sometimes an author may feel that the suggestions are unnecessary, lack appreciation of the work or are manufactured for the sake of writing something. As an author you have several routes open to you if you disagree with the comments made. You can write to the editor and appeal, you can write to the editor and explain why you are unable to make the requested revisions and negotiate a compromise, or you can do all that is asked of you in order to get published. How desperate the author is to publish and how much power the editor and reviewer wish to exert, will influence the decision that an author has to make.

As the 'gatekeepers of the academic community' (French, 1993b) the reviewer and editor hold the power to accept, reject, alter and shape knowledge. This power can mean that the process of selecting articles is sometimes unfair or biased. For example, reviewers may knowingly or unknowingly reject work that challenges their own ideas and writings or they may be biased towards one kind of methodology (usually quantitative in therapy research). French (1993b) offers reflections of her own experiences of the peer review system, which include a curt and disapproving review which shook her confidence, and being forced to remove contentious paragraphs.

No system that involves human judgement is going to be completely fair or unbiased, so authors will need to be prepared for a lengthy negotiation period in which they are assertive over the issues that are important within the study and never prejudice their principles. It may be sensible, however, to be conciliatory over small matters that are of less importance (French, 1993b; Brodie *et al.*, 1994).

Ethics and censorship

The ethics of dissemination and the possibility of censorship come into play when we think about the people that have a vested interest in the research. Ethical issues in dissemination include the areas of anonymity, confidentiality, copyright and accuracy of reporting. Robson (1993) notes that participants in the research may be concerned with how they are presented in a report. Participants often provide you with personal or confidential information on the understanding that they will not be identified in the report. Authors therefore need to ensure that they can honour any assurances of anonymity and confidentiality that they gave to research participants.

When an article is accepted for publication authors often have to sign a copyright agreement. This agreement will state that the work the author has written is original, has not been published elsewhere and is not the work of another person. The agreement will also outline who owns the copyright of the article once it is published. This will vary from journal to journal. Some journals will claim sole ownership of the article; others will outline a kind of 'joint ownership' in which authors can take copies of the articles for educational or research use. Authors often have to seek permission from the journal publishers to reproduce their article in another publication (for example, turning an article into a chapter in a book). Copyright issues often bring into question the ownership of research and can cause authors to become quite frustrated, so check the copyright agreement carefully before you sign.

In considering the reporting of results Glass (1994, p. 336) warns us that we have a duty to report the results of clinical trials accurately, because failure to do so may result in harm to patients:

> 'Responsibility for avoiding potential harm from inadequate disclosure touches other issues, such as complete and accurate reporting of efficacy criteria, side-effects, editorial decisions not to report negative findings, or even the way the data are structured for presentation'.

Censorship of dissemination may come into play if the sponsors of research have concerns regarding how they are portrayed in the report. They will be concerned with whether the report will be used by others to criticize or undermine them. In some cases sponsors of reports can stop you from disseminating results if they don't 'like' what you have written. Sponsors may not 'like' your report because it does not fit the current political climate or the current policies of the organization. Like copyright issues, censorship from sponsors brings into question the ownership of research.

Key points

1. There are four reasons why dissemination of research is important: so therapy can grow and develop, to contribute to the body of knowledge, so our ideas are critically analysed by other people and to contribute to the reduction of the gap between therapy and practice.
2. The reasons why researchers may fail to disseminate their work include: a fear of rejection, the additional time and energy required and assuming someone else will do it.
3. The five major methods of dissemination are: journal articles, conference abstracts, talks and presentations, posters and publications in the popular press.
4. The dissemination method you choose will depend on your target audience.
5. The purpose of the peer review system is to select articles and presentations that are of a suitable academic standard.
6. The peer review system is not completely fair or unbiased.
7. There are three main ethical issues regarding dissemination: anonymity and confidentiality, copyright and accuracy of reporting.
8. Sponsors of your research may wish to censor what you disseminate due to concern over how they are portrayed or the current political climate.

References

Ballinger, C., Curtin, M., Eakin, P., Hollis, V., Nicol, M. and Telford, R. (1996). Writing an abstract. *British Journal of Occupational Therapy*, **59,** 33–35.

Brodie, D.A., Williams, J.G. and Glynn Owens, R. (1994). *Research Methods for the Health Sciences.* Harwood Academic Publishers.

Chapman, J., Davey, C. and Seale, J. (1997). *Assessment conflict in a therapy degree: motivation to pass versus motivation to learn.* Paper presented to the Staff Education and Development Association Conference, Plymouth.

Cormack, D.F.S. (1994). *Writing for Health Care Professions.* Blackwell Scientific Publications.

Currier, D.P. (1990). *Elements of Research in Physiotherapy.* Williams and Wilkins.

Dickson, R. (1994). Dissemination and implementation: the wider picture. *Nurse Researcher*, **4**, 5–13.

French, S. (1993a). *Practical Research: A Guide for Therapists.* Butterworth-Heinemann.

French, S. (1993b). Telling. In *Reflecting on Research Practice.* (P. Shakespeare, D. Atkinson and S. French, eds), pp. 119–130. Open University Press.

Glass, K.C. (1994). Toward a duty to report clinical trials accurately: the clinical alert and beyond. *The Journal of Law, Medicine and Ethics*, **22**, 327–338.

Maykut, P. and Morehouse, R. (1996). *Beginning Qualitative Research: A Philosophic and Practical Guide.* The Falmer Press.

Robson, C. (1993). *Real World Research: A Resource for Social Scientists and Practitioner-Researchers.* Blackwell.

Complementary reading

Andrews, K. (1993). Writing for medical journals. *Clinical Rehabilitation*, **7**, 91–98.

Braddom, C.L. (1990). A framework for writing and/or evaluating papers. *American Journal of Physical Medicine and Rehabilitation*, **69**, 333–335.

Crosbie, J., Cole, J. and Galley, P. (1993). Promoting quality in the reporting of research. *Australian Journal of Physiotherapy*, **39**, 165–168.

Fowkes, F.G.R. and Fulton, P.M. (1991). Critical appraisal of published research: introductory guidelines. *British Medical Journal*, **302**, 1136–1140.

Harms, M. (1995). How to prepare a poster presentation. *Physiotherapy*, **81**, 276–277.

Lehmkuhl, L.D. (1987). Mixing one part common sense with each part statistics in planning the design and reporting the results of clinical research in physical therapy. *Physical Therapy*, **67**, 1851–1853.

Leininger, M. (1994). Evaluation criteria and critique of qualitative research studies. In *Critical Issues in Qualitative Research Methods.* (J.M. Morse, ed.). Sage Publications.

Richardson, A., Jackson, C. and Sykes, W. (1990). *Taking Research Seriously. Means of Improving and Assessing the Use and Dissemination of Research.* HMSO.

Walker, M. (1997). A survival guide to paper presentation. *British Journal of Occupational Therapy*, **60**, 26–28.

One step forwards or one step backwards?

The snakes and ladders of research

Any of you who have conducted a piece of research will probably agree that there were ups and downs, highs and lows during the course of your project. In this respect doing research is a bit like a game of snakes and ladders. Usually we try to avoid the 'snakes' of research before we start, but with the best will in the world, something is going to go wrong! It may be that you do not get enough questionnaires returned, the computer crashes and loses all your data, the interview you tape-recorded is inaudible, the ethics committee take too long to consider your proposal or the journal editor makes some negative comments about your paper. Whatever the nature of the 'snake' that you find on your research journey, it is likely to have an effect on your feelings about doing research. This effect may be short term or long term. You may decide you hate doing research and never want to do it again or you may decide to treat it as a lesson that you will learn from for next time.

Whilst the 'snakes' of research can be upsetting and demoralizing, it is important to view them alongside the 'ladders' of research. Usually we conduct research with the expectation of climbing certain 'ladders', such as improving your career prospects or gaining recognition from your peers. However, just as some 'snakes' can be unexpected so can some 'ladders'. For example, you may feel surprised at the feeling of accomplishment you experience when you finish your project or revel in the prospect of influencing other people's work and ideas.

This chapter will highlight in more detail the potential costs and benefits of undertaking research and how these may influence the lessons you learn from research and the decisions you make about where to go to next.

The costs of undertaking research

If you are conducting a publicly funded piece of research then it is likely that one of the major down sides of being involved in such research is going to be the external pressures placed upon you. These pressures may involve finishing the work on time, producing regular reports, attending frequent steering committees and staying within budget. If you can survive these pressures then your standing in the research community may improve as you establish a 'name for yourself'. However, as Frost and Stablein (1992, p. 277) warn, the effort required in surviving these pressures may affect the quality of your work and your personal life:

> 'We worry about what these time constraints do to the quality of research in the field as well as the quality of the lives of the researchers themselves. We worry about increasing amounts of research done mindlessly and frantically, as researchers find themselves in an activity trap, chasing knowledge to meet extrinsic pressures'.

If the findings from your research are not what you expected or do not support your hypothesis you may experience a strong emotional response, particularly if the research is close to your heart or you have invested a lot of time and energy in the project. You may respond with feelings of surprise, shock, depression or denial. Whatever your response, it may be heavily influenced by a desire not to look a fool or a failure. Researchers faced with this crisis have been known to tamper with the data or change the hypothesis to fit the data. The simple advice for those experiencing this dilemma is that all results tell us something, even those we are not expecting. Sometimes such advice will be hard to take. But perhaps a good researcher is one who is open to the discovery of the unexpected.

Researchers often face 'issues of conscience' during the course of their research, which can make the research experience a painful one. For example, there may be a temptation to omit some of the steps of gaining informed consent in order to guarantee that you get the expected number of participants. It is not uncommon for interview or observation participants to divulge information (unrelated to the project) which the researcher feels should be related to authorities such as social or health care workers, were it not for the issue of confidentiality. A researcher may come under pressure from a sponsor to alter the slant of a report so as not to show a product or an organization in a 'bad light'. Pressures such as time and funding may tempt a researcher to collect data before formal ethical approval has been received. All these dilemmas might seem to have obvious solutions to the impartial bystander but can cause a great amount of guilt and anxiety for those researchers caught in the middle of the dilemma. A researcher caught in an 'ethical dilemma' should be able to seek advice from a supervisor or a colleague, but they must take some degree of responsibility for whatever decision they make following that advice.

The benefits of undertaking research

In Chapter 1 we discussed how the occupational therapy and physiotherapy professions would benefit from research because it would raise their professional status, give them ownership of their own knowledge-base and provide evidence upon which practice can be based. This is all true of course; however, very few of us undertake research without expecting there to be some personal benefits for ourselves.

Some personal benefits of undertaking research are tangible and immediate, others are less tangible and less immediate. Obvious tangible benefits of conducting research might include obtaining a qualification or promotion. Less obvious benefits are those such as having the opportunity to travel around and meet interesting people in the process of collecting data, having access to specialized equipment or having a break from clinical work. Other benefits for yourself may include having the freedom and space to think and be creative or being in control of your timetable. On completion of a research project you may gain benefits in terms of a boost to your pride, feelings of accomplishment and self-confidence.

Depending on the nature of your study, the people who took part in your study may also gain some benefit from your results and be able to use them to their advantage. For example, in her study of computer use in nine adult training centres, Seale (1993) provided each centre with a report of her findings. Some of the feedback she received suggested that some staff and managers had found her involvement beneficial because it helped to inform their decisions about future work and plans.

What have I learnt?   In evaluating your research experience you will probably weigh up the costs and the benefits of conducting your project and draw conclusions about what you have learnt from conducting the research. All researchers, from undergraduate students to research fellows, need to be able to draw lessons from their research that will enable them to improve on their techniques and methods in future work. The following quotes from undergraduate dissertations help to highlight some common lessons regarding the design of questionnaires and the piloting of interviews.

Padfield (1997, p. 44) conducted a questionnaire survey of carers of relatives with dementia in order to obtain their experiences of having attended a carer support group:

> 'The high ratings for all aspects of the support group evaluation raises a question over the sensitivity of the evaluation tool and whether the carers were worried about losing their support group if they responded negatively. More viable results may have been obtained if questions had been expanded to see exactly what worries had been dealt with and what sessions were of relevance to the carers'.

Connolly (1996, p. 55) interviewed carers of elderly relatives who needed respite care:

> 'In hindsight a pilot study of the interview would have been useful in allowing changes in some of the questions. Some questions during the interview needed to be rephrased so that the carer was able to understand what the author meant. It would also have given a better indication of the time required to conduct the interview'.

Our experience as supervisors is that it is sometimes hard to convince students that there is no such thing as 'a perfect research project' and that it is not an admission of failure to outline how you would improve things if you were to conduct the project again. For example, another student (Gibson, 1996, p. 54) conducted a study to compare the job satisfaction levels of physiotherapists working in elderly care and outpatients. She concluded that:

> 'Job satisfaction has been stated as a continuous adaptation between individuals and their work environment. It is therefore recommended that a longitudinal study or a test–retest design be used to document individual perceptions over a period of time, providing a more reliable and accurate picture of respondents job satisfaction'.

Perhaps one of the most important lessons for all of us to learn about research is that it is not a flawless process. Frost and Stablein (1992, p. 290) suggest that we need to be freed from the 'tyranny of having to match the ideal image of research as an orderly, trouble free and unemotional undertaking'.

Conducting research may help you 'learn by doing' and improve your understanding of the research process, but it may also help you learn more about yourself and how you feel about research. Conducting research may help you learn about yourself by giving you a greater insight into the skills that you possess or your ability to transfer skills across different situations. For example, conducting research tests your communication, persuasion, negotiation, organization, analysis and presentation skills, as well as many others. People will react to their research experiences in different ways. Some of us will decide that we love research, some of us will decide that we hate it. Some of our reactions may surprise us. For example, students often embark on their projects expecting that they are going to hate it and are quite surprised when they find that, for the most part, they enjoyed their experience. On the other hand, it is not unknown for PhD students to be terribly disappointed by their experiences and feel that it was one huge anticlimax. Whatever our personal reactions are to our research experiences, they will strongly influence our decisions about what to do next.

Where do I go from here?

After reflecting on the costs and benefits of being involved in the collection and analysis of research data and deciding on what you have learnt from the whole process, you are likely to make decisions about whether you want to conduct some more research or give it all up. If you decide that you want to conduct some more research then there are various options open to you, depending on whether you want to live in the academic or clinical world. You can register for a Masters or a PhD, you can apply for a research post in someone else's project, you can try to gain funds to run your own project or you can supervise an undergraduate or postgraduate project.

Given that we have written a book, which for the most part has tried to persuade you to see the importance of research, you may find what we say next strange. If, after your first experience of conducting research, you want to give it up, fine, give it up; don't take that one step forward into the 'front line'. However, making the decision not to collect and analyse data yourself does not necessarily mean that you are taking a regressive step backwards or that you have to leave the research world altogether. There are people in the research world other than those who collect and analyse data. It is argued that all therapists have a responsibility to critique and implement research findings. Some therapists will be responsible for funding and commissioning research and there is an important group of people who help others to conduct research projects. That help may come in the shape of distributing questionnaires on behalf of a student, brainstorming ideas with a colleague, allowing staff time off work, arranging for staff training and so on. Whatever role you choose to play, it is probably fair to say that you will not be able to avoid thinking about research in some guise or other. To use a financial analogy, you still have to pay tax regardless of whether it is you, your accountant or the taxman who calculates it! What we hope is that this book enables your thinking about the roles you want take in research to be informed.

Key points

1. There are both costs and benefits in conducting research.
2. Conducting research may improve your understanding of the research process and help you learn more about yourself and how you feel about research.
3. There are many roles to be filled in the research world other than that of data gatherer.

References

Connolly, N. (1996). *Respite care: are the needs of carers of elderly relatives being met?* Third year dissertation, School of Occupational Therapy and Physiotherapy, University of Southampton.

Frost, P. and Stablein, R. (1992). *Doing Exemplary Research.* Sage Publications.

Gibson, S. (1996). *Job satisfaction of physiotherapists in elderly care and outpatients: is there a difference?* Third year dissertation, School of Occupational Therapy and Physiotherapy, University of Southampton.

Hignett, S. (1994). Research snakes and ladders. *Therapy Weekly*, **3 Feb.**, 7.

Padfield, S. (1997). *Carers of relatives with dementia – their experiences, feelings and perceptions of having attended a carer support group.* Third year dissertation, School of Occupational Therapy and Physiotherapy, University of Southampton.

Seale, J. (1993). *Microcomputers in adult special education: the management of innovation*, PhD thesis (2 volumes), University of Keele.

Answers to exercises

Some of the exercises given in this book do not have set answers that can easily be identified as right or wrong. In this section answers will be provided for exercises where the authors feel advice or guidance on the kinds of answers or solutions that can be derived would be useful.

Chapter 2

Exercise: Finding the scope of the topic

One way of approaching this task is to try and identify some key words that you can use to search for relevant literature. For example, if we take the Roberta Adams example, three possible key words might spring to mind: rheumatoid arthritis, physiotherapy and patient education. A BIDS Embase (computerized literature data base) search on each of these key words reveals the following number of 'hits' in terms of articles found that were published in 1997:

- Rheumatoid arthritis – 2031 hits.
- Patient education – 978 hits.
- Physiotherapy – 851 hits.

Getting Embase to list all 2031 articles related to rheumatoid arthritis on the screen is probably not going to be helpful; you need to narrow the search. Combining key words can do this. For example, conducting a combined search for rheumatoid arthritis *and* patient education revealed 20 hits, one of which was an article that sounded quite interesting:

Lindroth, Y. *et al.* (1997). A problem-based education program for patients with rheumatoid arthritis. Evaluation after three and twelve months. *Arthritis Care Research*, **10**, 325–332.

Don't forget to check whether the system you are using has other key words that might be used instead of the key words you have chosen. For example, a Thesaurus search in BIDS Embase revealed the following associated terms for rheumatoid arthritis:

- Arthritis deformans.
- Chronic polyarthritis.
- Chronic rheumatoid arthritis.
- Infantile rheumatoid arthritis.

Table A.1   A possible coding scheme for questions 3, 4, 5 and 9

Question	Response	Code
Question 3	Occupational therapist	1
	Physiotherapist	2
Question 4	None	1
	0–5 years	2
	5+ years	3
Question 5	Take sole responsibility for supervision	1
	Supervise jointly with a colleague	2
	Supervise first years only	3
	Supervise second years only	4
	Supervise third years only	5
	Supervise students at any level	6
	Supervise one student at a time	7
	Supervise more than one student at a time	8
Question 9	Strongly agree	5
	Agree	4
	Neither agree or disagree	3
	Disagree	2
	Strongly disagree	1

Chapter 4

Exercise: Supervising and grading students on clinical/fieldwork placement questionnaire

Questions 3 and 4 are dichotomous questions. Question 5 is a check-list question. Question 8 is an open question and question 9 is a scaled question. Questions 7 and 9 attempt to check the consistency of response regarding the ease of grading. (See Table A.1 for a possible coding scheme for questions 3, 4, 5 and 9.)

The questionnaire could be improved by altering the band areas for question 4. If someone has no experience of supervising students, it is feasible that they could tick the 'none' box or the '0–5' box. If someone has 5 years' supervising experience they may tick the '0–5' or the '5+' box. It may be helpful to ask respondents to explain their ratings for questions 6, 7 and 9. Finally, the open questions do not allow a lot of space for respondents to write.

Chapter 6

Exercise: Definitions of categories

One of the problems of creating observation categories is that you have to be very explicit about the definitions you attach to them. In the example given there is a distinction between engagement with staff, patients and visitors, but what does engagement mean? Did you and your colleagues come up with similar definitions? There are a number of behaviours that might be considered indicative of 'engage-ment'. Behaviours indicative of verbal engagement might include laughing, talking, shouting, asking and answering questions and crying. Behaviours indicative of non-verbal engagement might include eye contact, gestures (for help or attention), physical presence (sitting by the bed or chair), touch (cuddles, pats, strokes) and facial expressions.

Chapter 9

Exercise: Research activity data

Ranking the research activities in order from lowest mean (most likely to engage in) to highest mean (least likely to engage in) reveals that therapy students think doctors are more likely than therapists to speak at conferences, analyse clinical data, publish research articles and be independent researchers (see Figure A.1). While the data show some similarities in rankings, a closer inspection of the differences between the means reveals some interesting findings. For example, generating research ideas is ranked the seventh most likely behaviour for both therapists and doctors. Therapy students, however, consider that therapists are slightly less likely to do this (mean $= 2.95$) than doctors (mean $= 2.52$).

The mean may be considered the most useful average to use because it is more likely to reveal differences than the median and the mode. If you check back to the original table in Chapter 9, the median and mode are often the same for both groups. However, one may need to question how meaningful the mean is with its decimal places, when it has been derived from numbers that have been nominally assigned to categories such as highly probable and most unlikely.

The information from the ranges reveals that, for all but one statement, responses ranged from 1 to 5 for therapists and doctors. Thus, there was a wide variation in responses. An examination of the standard deviations reveals that for all the statements there was a wider variation for the statements regarding doctors than those regarding therapists. Therapy students were slightly less consistent in their responses regarding doctors. A comparison of the differences

Therapists:	Doctors:
1. Reading research journal articles	1. Reading research journal articles
1. Attending conferences and workshops	1. Attending conferences and workshops
2. Applying research findings to practice	2. Applying research findings to practice
3. Reading non-research journal articles	3. Speaking at conferences and workshops
4. Collecting clinical data	4. Analysing clinical data
5. Analysing clinical data	5. Reading non-research journal articles
6. Speaking at conferences and workshops	6. Collecting clinical data
7. Generating research ideas	7. Generating research ideas
8. Being a research assistant or collaborator	8. Publishing research articles
9. Publishing non-research articles	9. Being an independent or principal researcher
10. Publishing research articles	10. Publishing non-research articles
11. Being an independent or principal researcher	11. Being a research assistant or collaborator

Figure A.1   Ranking of research activity statements from most likely to least likely.

between the means and the differences between the standard deviations reveals that the two statements that have the largest differences between their means (publishing non-research articles and publishing research articles) also have large differences between their standard deviations. The difference in variations suggests that it may be unwise to make much of the difference in means for these two statements.

Information regarding means and standard deviations could be presented using a bar chart, with different colour bars representing therapist and doctor. Information regarding reasons behind the ratings would be useful in order to gain a wider understanding of the results presented. For example, why do therapy students think doctors are more likely than therapists to speak at conferences, analyse clinical data, publish research articles and be independent researchers?

Chapter 14

Exercise: Ranking of ethical scenarios

When we give the four scenarios to our students they tend to rank scenario 4 as the one that causes them most concern, followed by scenarios 3 and 2. Scenario 1 causes them the least concern. How do these rankings compare to your rankings? If we examine the scenarios in a little more detail, these rankings become quite interesting.

Scenario 4 probably raises most concern because it involves a vulnerable group of people, adults with severe learning difficulties. The concern is centred on the two issues of 'covert' filming and whether the residential manager had any 'right' to give consent on behalf of his client group. Getting informed consent from people with severe learning disabilities can be difficult if they cannot read information sheets, cannot easily comprehend verbal communication or have difficulties communicating their understanding. With this in mind, it is not unusual or unethical for parents or guardians to give consent on behalf of those they are caring for. However, what might be considered unethical is giving consent for such an 'invasive' data collection technique, particularly when the data could be collected by other means such as overt observations from known observers.

Scenario 3 raises two issues concerning whether it is ethical to use risky or untested drugs and treatments in research trials and methods of contacting potential participants. Using untried treatments is only unethical if the participants are not given enough information to enable them to give full informed consent. A possible concern about contacting women at high risk of developing breast cancer is that they may not know that they are considered high risk, so great care would need to be taken in choosing and approaching potential participants.

Scenario 2 initially raises issues about paying participants to take part in studies. On the one hand, payments can be considered coercive, while on the other hand, they can be considered just compensation for the time that someone gives to take part in a study. If someone is paid to take part in a research study they may feel obliged to participate even when they would prefer not to. This can be a problem if half-way through a study the participant become uneasy, distressed or alarmed at what they are being asked to do. Their gut instinct may be to leave, but they may feel that they cannot because they have been paid to stay until the end. Studies in which payments are offered as inducements to participate need to create a clear procedure for informed consent in which participants know that they can leave at any time even though they have been paid.

Scenario 1 probably raises least ethical concern because it does not involve a vulnerable group of people. However, it does raise issues concerning professional behaviour. There is a strong case for arguing that the researcher in this scenario has abused and wasted the therapists' time if he has no intention of using or publishing the outcomes. In addition, the failure of the researcher to inform the therapists of his intentions regarding the data indicates a lack of respect for the therapists. If we were one of those therapists we would feel terribly 'used' and would probably refuse to take part in any other study ever again. While this decision may not have an impact on the original researcher it will have a huge impact on any future researchers who dare to step into that particular outpatients department!

Chapter 15

Exercise: critiquing a research proposal

A précis of the proposal might look like this:

OT and PT students at x University spend 38 weeks of the three-year course on clinical placement supervised and assessed by clinicians (clinical/fieldwork supervisors). There is a need to offer supervisors a consistent approach to student assessment and measure the reliability of performance gradings. This will be done by devising case studies representing a range of student abilities that will be assessed by 10 lecturing staff to test inter-rater reliability. The five most consistent studies will form the basis of an evaluated briefing exercise with supervisors. Data will be analysed statistically using SPSS.

This project is probably achievable with co-operation and well researched, careful development of the case studies.

Index